P rescribed Pilates
for Pain Management

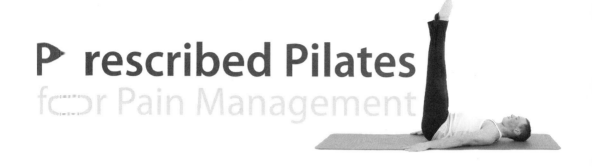

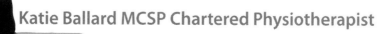

Katie Ballard MCSP Chartered Physiotherapist

Published by
KTB Publishers Limited
1st Floor Westgate House
Spital Street
Dartford
DA1 2EH
www.pilatesandtherapy.co.uk

KTB Prescribed Pilates is a registered trademark

ISBN: 978-0-9557717-0-5

Photography
www.clivewoodleyphotography.co.uk

Models
Laura Hills   Dancer / Model
Liam Durbidge   World and British Number One Junior Acrobatic Gymnast

Designed by
David Tokeley

Acknowledgments

There are so many people to thank for making this book come together.

To my husband, Toby, for his continued belief in me and ongoing support throughout the development of KTB. Without you my dream would not have been made possible. To my parents who are always there for me. Thanks Mom for all those Sunday roasts that kept me going during the long Sundays of writing. My thanks also to my admin team for their enthusiasm and support during this project. David, thank you for your hard work with our tight deadline. Clive, thank you for the photography.

An important thank you must go to Jane Simmonds, lecturer at the University of Hertfordshire and my licensed physical therapist. You were the one who picked me up when I needed guidance and gave me the interest in core stability from the start. I know you will still put me back on the right road when I need further advice. Thank you for being there for me.

I must also say a big thank you to all our clients who loyally followed us when we moved to our bigger studios and who spread the word of the work we are doing. I am grateful for your support, loyalty and often friendship.

Contents

Chapter 5: Understanding & Working through the Assessment Exercises

Chapter 6: Rehabilitation Exercises

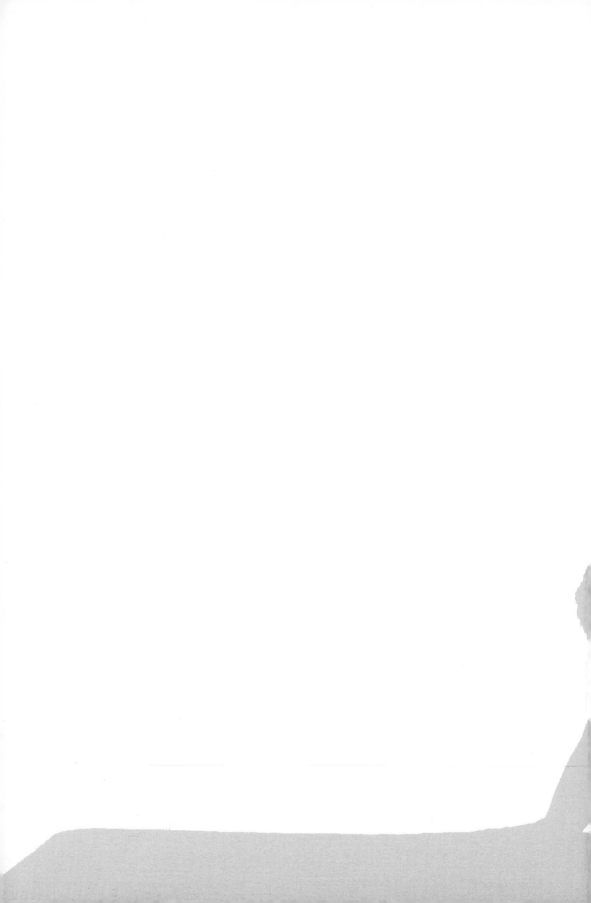

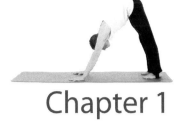

Chapter 1
Introducing the Author—Katie Ballard MSPT

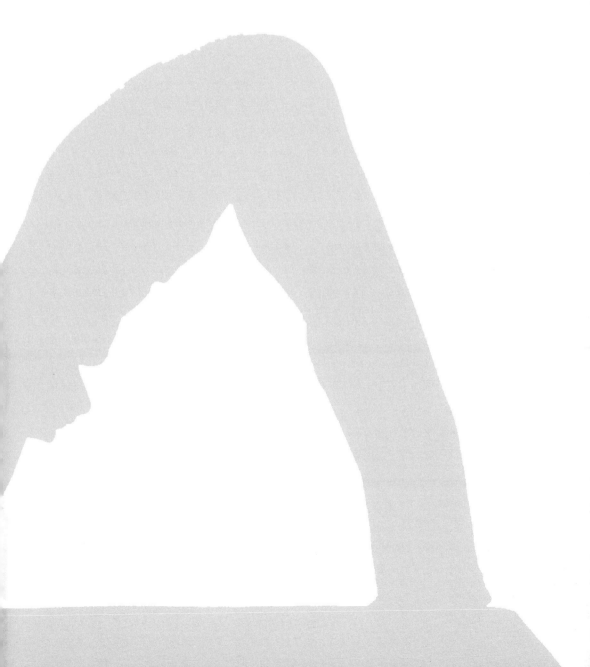

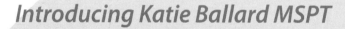

Introducing Katie Ballard MSPT

Katie Ballard developed Prescribed Pilates so that she could share her experience of using Pilates to improve health, increase postural awareness and reduce pain. Pilates was designed for rehabilitation and that is why many individuals start Prescribed Pilates following a sports injury, for chronic spinal pain, improvement of posture or simply to gain confidence in exercise.

The success of Prescribed Pilates can partly be attributed to Katie's ability to empathize with her patients, bringing understanding of pain management and working to change lifestyles in order to reduce symptoms. Katie has a rheumatology condition that was diagnosed while she was studying for her physical therapy degree. This collagen disorder meant Katie suffered pain throughout her physical therapy training after forcing her to give up county standard athletics (equivalent to state standards here in the U.S.) and swimming in her teens. Despite consulting various

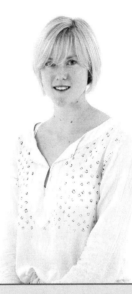

specialists, from a young age Katie failed to receive guidance on how she could help herself and received no answers on what to expect in the future. Frustrated with the lack of ongoing support and with being advised to leave her physical therapy degree, Katie finally found guidance from a physical therapist who had a similar condition to herself. Inspired that a future career in physical therapy was realistic, Katie began a rehabilitation program of core stability and gentle muscle building exercise. After dedicating six months solely to improving posture, making progress with her exercises and changing her whole way of life, Katie became stronger and gained control over her pain. She was then ready to complete her degree and graduate as a certified physical therapist. Early in her career Katie specialized her physical therapy practice toward therapeutic exercise and Pilates, knowing from personal experience that this was the area in which she could have the most impact to understand and assist her patients. Katie now gains enormous satisfaction in helping patients to develop awareness of their pain and in supporting them to take control of their rehabilitation and lifestyle change. She is proud to present her teachings, understanding and exercise classifications in this, her first book *Prescribed Pilates*.

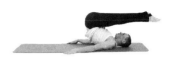

Chapter 2

What Is Pilates?

Pilates is more than an exercise regime, it teaches a new way of using your body, increasing postural awareness and the way in which you perform your daily activities.

One of the main benefits of Pilates, from a physical therapist's perspective, is that the technique can be successful in correcting muscle imbalances. These imbalances are caused by us overusing certain muscles while others are neglected and become weak. Muscle imbalance is a recognized source of pain and often leads to a reduced performance in a sporting or everyday activity. Pilates will help you to understand where these muscle imbalances may be developing and how you can correct them. It is therefore a self-management technique for reducing pain and improving the performance of any task. Many people today have poor posture leading to the spine becoming curved. This curvature will throw the spine out of natural alignment, reducing flexibility and causing pain. The Pilates approach will improve flexibility, correct postural dysfunctions and therefore ease pain caused by poor posture. It is a technique that is promoted by physical therapists, Osteopaths and GPs and is rapidly gaining recognition within the celebrity and elite sports world.

Although Pilates has recently enjoyed increased publicity, it is not a new technique; the first Pilates studio was opened in 1926 in New York by Joseph Pilates. Joseph himself said, "People won't understand the brilliance of my work for 50 years" and he was right. That quote was made about 50 years ago!

The History of Joseph Pilates

Joseph Humbertus Pilates, born in Germany, was a frail child who suffered from rickets, asthma and rheumatic fever. Joseph was devoted to overcoming his ailments and he achieved this by combining Eastern disciplines of yoga and martial arts with Western forms of physical activities such as bodybuilding, gymnastics, boxing and recreational sports. He did this so well that by the age of fourteen he had perfected his physique and was asked to model for anatomical charts! In 1912 Joseph moved to England where he became a circus performer and boxer and worked as a self-defense trainer for detectives at Scotland Yard. When World War I broke out, Joseph was interned as a prisoner of war. He taught his exercise regime, now called Contrology, to his fellow detainees. Interestingly, those who had followed Joseph's Contrology survived the 1918 influenza epidemic. This survival was attributed to the physically enhanced lung capacity gained from Pilates exercises. Joseph was then sent to the Isle of Man where he was trained as a nurse orderly to care for those wounded in the war. The traditional matwork exercises were now inappropriate for this kind of population. Joseph responded to this change of client by designing apparatus that could turn hospital beds into resistance rehabilitation equipment using the springs of the beds. This succeeded in returning the soldiers to full fitness whatever their injury. After the end of the war, Joseph decided to move to America, en route meeting his future wife, Clara, a nurse with a shared interest in restoring others to health. On reaching America they set up their fitness studio in New York and over the next forty years Joseph continued to use Contrology to rehabilitate dancers, athletes, acrobats and entertainers and to maintain the extreme physical fitness their bodies needed, correcting any problems they faced. In 1967 Joseph sadly passed away, leaving his techniques to be taught by his students.

Pilates Today

In the Sports World

Today, Pilates is no longer the secret of elite dancers, though it is used commonly by many top dance centers. As many high profile celebrities come from a dance background, the appreciation of the benefits of the Pilates method has reached the famous and, subsequently, the media. Celebrities have increased the profile of Pilates and have sent figures attending classes soaring. The general sports world is now beginning to acknowledge the advantages of using the Pilates approach to build strength without excess bulk, increase body awareness, and improve flexibility, agility and economy of motion. Premier football clubs consult with Pilates instructors to incorporate exercises into their training, top professional rugby clubs use Pilates to improve flexibility and many elite sports performers use Pilates for injury prevention.

In the Healthcare World

Clinical Pilates classes are more frequently being taken within physical therapy departments nationwide. Evidence-based practice is something that medical practitioners and allied health professionals, including physical therapists, must adhere to in both the National Health Service (NHS) and the private sector when treating patients. Guidelines for treatment are set, based on this evidence. Current guidelines set within Europe state that correcting muscle imbalance, exercise and education of lifestyle changes are important within the management of low back pain. Pilates is one technique that will address this and is therefore accepted within the remedial world to improve spinal pain, rehabilitate joint injury and prevent recurrence of these problems. Physical therapy-led Pilates classes are becoming more frequently seen within physical therapy practices and in the community. These classes provide health professionals with a safe outlet where they can refer their patients for continued rehabilitation after discharge, under the guidance of a trained professional.

In the Gym World

Pilates is also becoming more common in the gym environment. Some call this Fitness Pilates. These sessions are great for giving diversity to the usual gym-based routines that typically require aerobic endurance, impact and resistance in the form of weights. The problem, however, is that such regimes are not usually appropriate for anyone with an existing injury. These sessions will not typically give an adequate explanation as to what the Pilates approach tries to achieve, making it difficult to gain functional carry-over from these classes, as they are not taught in a way which will improve the execution of our activities of daily living. Posture too frequently remains unchanged by attending these classes, as the individual is often not given enough attention and class members are not assessed individually. These classes are taught more generically and at a mixed ability level.

Pilates Isn't Easy!

Pilates is not easy at first, but what is? Think back to when you first learned to drive. The first thing you had to do on your first lesson was to sit in the car and familiarize yourself with the different pedals, switches and dials. In Pilates, this is the equivalent to learning how the posture should be; what is neutral spine? How do you activate the transversus muscle to 30 percent? How does it feel to soften the ribs and relax the shoulders? Back to your driving lesson: before you are asked to negotiate a busy freeway you will be taken along quiet roads, where there is less chance of meeting another car. You will now have to remember how to control the car and move forward at the same time. In Pilates you will start with level one exercises—gentle movements that require less coordination or strength than later movements but still require you to maintain your correct posture. As you get better with your driving, with more practice, your instructor will take you onto busier roads, you will drive at busier times and you will negotiate more complex situations. It is the same with Pilates; once you have learned to control the lower level exercises, you will try the more intermediate and then advanced movements. Ultimately, as the control becomes more automatic, you will be able to apply the posture you have learned to your functional tasks without inhibiting and actually improving that task. When you next get into your car, you will instinctively know what to do, without thinking about which pedal is the accelerator. You could also apply the knowledge you have of driving to another car if you were to rent one while on holiday. Pilates is the same; it is just another motor task that you have learned. As with any new skill, the more you practice the more it will become automatic. I strongly believe, however, that to practice and gain this automatic response you need an understanding of how the technique works. This reinforces the importance of a structured class and a knowledgeable instructor.

Pilates and Breathing

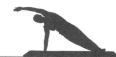

It was believed that the improved fitness of the lungs achieved through Pilates exercises was what helped prevent the soldiers in the prisoner-of-war camps from contracting the influenza virus that killed so many during World War I. Breathing in Pilates involves expanding the lower rib cage outwards during inhalation. The shoulders will remain relaxed. Research shows us that the "in" breath helps the diaphragm to stabilize the trunk, and the exhalation helps to execute better movement. Many of us cannot perform some of the more advanced movements unless we get the breathing right. Functionally, if you can control the breath, everyday tasks will be performed with less effort and more control. Many beginners struggle with breathing. The simple rule is to breathe out with a movement away from the body, or when you need more control. It is also important to practice the breathing functionally. The more you try to expand and empty the lungs using this lateral breathing, the easier it will become. As you improve you will begin to appreciate the importance of the breath. Initially, please don't let it put you off the exercises.

Pilates Is a Mind-Body Technique

Pilates is different from other forms of exercise, in that it requires you to think about the movements that you are doing and where the movement is coming from. The use of imagery helps to establish this mind-body connection and allows you to understand how the movements should be executed. For example, if you are imagining eggshells under the feet, your brain will tell your body to lighten the pressure under your feet. If you are imagining a helium balloon lifting the back of the head, then when walking, your brain will tell the back of the head to lightly lift up to allow your posture to become more upright. It is important that you think about every movement so that you understand where you should be moving from (your tummy, the central core of stability) and where, in fact, you are moving from, which may not be correct. If your brain remains unaware of the differences, then you will not be able to change the way in which the movement is performed and the movement will remain unchanged. Once the control has been improved on the mat you will be ready to apply this new control into functional movements. At first you may only be aware of what you may be doing wrong, but this is a great start. Once this has been acknowledged, you will start to focus on what you should be doing and you will then start to move differently. For example, in your first class you will be taught the correct position of the shoulders and rib cage and you will feel how different this may be to how your shoulders usually feel. Throughout the week before your next class, you will become aware of how often your shoulders tense and how you roll your shoulders forward whenever you move your arm. In the next session you will try harder to correct your shoulders, then in the next week you will focus on correcting the shoulders functionally, for example while brushing your teeth or combing your hair. If the brain is unaware of how the shoulders should feel when they are in the right position, you will not be aware of when they are wrong. It will not happen subconsciously for a long time, but with practice it will get better. The conscious change is the first major step for improvement.

Pilates and the Powerhouse

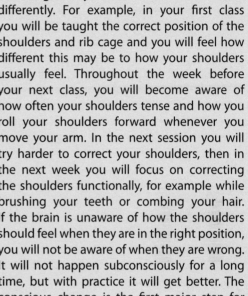

The powerhouse in Pilates is the area below the navel that wraps around the back acting like a corset to support the back during movement. Controlled by the deep abdominal muscle (the Transversus Abdominus), the Pelvic Floor, the Diaphragm and the Multifidus muscle in the back, these muscles activate at low intensities and support the back during movement. For numerous reasons including poor posture, a history of a back injury or following pregnancy, the ability of these muscles to protect has been reduced. Pilates will re-educate the body on how to use this powerhouse and how to strengthen the back. With this newly regained strength, you will be able to slowly reclaim the movement you once had and will be able to return to the functional activities that you may have stopped. You will learn more about the powerhouse in the spinal stability section of this book.

Joseph Pilates said that "in ten sessions you will feel the difference of Pilates; in twenty you will see the difference and in thirty you'll have a whole new body. So let's continue!"

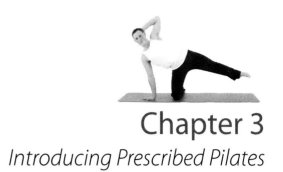

Chapter 3
Introducing Prescribed Pilates

Introducing Prescribed Pilates

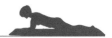

Joseph Pilates used his exercises, known as Contrology, to rehabilitate individuals after injury, working both with soldiers during World War I and from his New York studio after 1926. The success Pilates' teaching has in rehabilitation differentiates it from other forms of exercise and links it with physical therapy practice. Prescribed Pilates was developed by Katie Ballard, a certified physical therapist. It uses Pilates to increase postural awareness and to alter faulty patterns of movement by addressing muscle imbalances. Prescribed Pilates classifies its repertoire of exercises into four subgroups: **Spinal Stability, Pelvic Stability, Scapular Stability** and **Mobility**. Each of these areas need to be perfected in order to achieve good, safe execution of Joseph Pilates' original matwork exercises. Clinically, control in each of these areas leads to improved posture, inner strength, better balance and overall healthy movement, minimizing stress to the joints during everyday activities.

Current Pilates Teaching

Following the death of Joseph Pilates in 1967, the Pilates method has branched into two separate directions; the first is the Classical Pilates. This approach closely follows the teachings of Joseph Pilates himself and is good for rehabilitating and training at advanced levels, but is often too advanced for the general population or those needing rehabilitation. If performed incorrectly, this approach can actually cause more harm than good. The physical therapy approach, however, is much safer and is appropriate for any level of fitness and is advised for people with back pain or injury. The problem with clinical Pilates is that it can appear boring if it is not adequately explained and understood. Many people simply give up with the technique as they do not appreciate how working with small movements at low levels can be beneficial. Realistically, everybody needs to begin with the lower levels in order to understand the main principles and then you can advance safely. A problem with Pilates is that many people do not understand how to make progress, or cannot see the link between exercises. People also often do not understand what the exercises are trying to improve. Typically, we see people either pushing too hard to try to achieve a classic movement, or simply staying within their comfort zone by settling with the basic movements. Unfortunately, either way you will not be achieving the most from the Pilates method. In order for Pilates to give maximum benefit it must be understood. Prescribed Pilates is a way of categorizing the exercises so that you understand what they aim to achieve, you are aware of the focus points of each exercise and you are able to make progress from the movements. It helps you to understand the Pilates exercises and method and, importantly, make Pilates appropriate to your needs.

How Prescribed Pilates Differs from the Current Teaching Methods

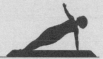

Prescribed Pilates is an approach that allows you to understand how correcting one exercise will enable you to move on to a more difficult movement. You will be working toward the original Contrology examples, but without having to achieve this advanced level. If you understand the requirements of each exercise, then you will start to understand which components you may be struggling with. You can then select the exercises that you need to improve to address these areas. You will soon find that achieving higher levels becomes easier and makes more sense. Throughout this learning experience you will become more and more aware of your body and will start to understand why certain daily activities may be causing you pain, or how particular movements, either within sport or your daily life, may be improved through Pilates. This method of Pilates' teaching puts you in control of your abilities and enables you to achieve the most from the Pilates approach both through exercise and functional postural changes.

Prescribed Pilates understands that individuals will find different aspects of each exercise difficult. If mobility is your weakest area, no matter how much abdominal strength training you do, you will still not be able to control the advanced movements until you have improved flexibility. It is necessary, therefore, to give each individual the most beneficial exercises from the Pilates repertoire to help them as individuals. The way that Prescribed Pilates is broken down makes it easy for each person to assess their area of weakness and work on correcting this.

Prescribed Pilates will benefit everyone whether you are working at a beginner, intermediate or advanced level. The only difference will be your starting point and the level that you are ultimately hoping to achieve. An imbalance or weakness in any of these areas could lead to, or could be contributing to, any pain or injuries that you may have. Identifying these areas through Prescribed Pilates allows you to rehabilitate, exercise and move in the most effective way for you.

Using This Book and Understanding the Prescribed Pilates Categorization

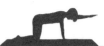

How to Use this Text

The exercises or movements of the Prescribed Pilates repertoire are divided into three chapters in this book. The first is the assessment exercises, then the rehabilitation exercises and finally the original advanced Contrology exercises.

Prescribed Pilates categorizes its repertoire of exercises into four sub-sections, these are

1. **Spinal Stability**—or lower abdominal strength

2. **Pelvic Stability**—or rotary control

3. **Scapular Stability**—or shoulder blade control

4. **Mobility**—or flexibility

All three chapters will divide the exercises into these four sections to aid understanding and progression.

Assessment

Before you begin with the rehabilitation exercises of each section, you need to read and understand all the assessment movements in this chapter, not only those from the relevant section. The assessment chapter will include a foreword for each subsection. This will explain the importance of perfecting the movements in each category, giving examples from a physical therapist's clinical perspective. The explanations given with each movement will make you aware of, and understand, what you need to concentrate on for the exercises in each category. As long as you think about what you are doing, you will understand when you are doing the exercise correctly and when the exercise may be too hard for you. From this, you will identify your starting level.

The Rehabilitation Exercises

After the assessment section, you will work through these rehabilitation exercises; they include beginning to advanced movements but the link between exercises is stated. There will also be links between the groups. It is important to note that there will be overlaps and the groups are not independent of one another. You will probably notice that some of the exercises in some groups are easier than others; generally it is the more difficult movements that you need to be practicing, as long as you are safe.

For each exercise, you will be made aware of:
1. The physical benefits of that exercise
2. Whether it is important to have perfected an easier movement prior to moving to this exercise
3. Any particular areas of concern that you will need to be aware of, if any
4. Modifications to make the exercise easier
5. Progressions to make the exercise harder
6. The exercise or series that you will be able to move onto once this exercise has been corrected

Original Contrology

These are the exercises from Josephs Pilates' original Contrology matwork program. They demonstrate the movements that require advanced control of the section you are working in, e.g. mobility, strength, pelvic control or scapular control. These are advanced movements and you will need control in all areas to be able to attempt these movements. It is helpful to understand these movements but not necessary to achieve perfect execution of them. These exercises are typically seen more within classical Pilates teaching.

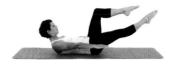

Chapter 4
Introducing the Four Sections of Prescribed Pilates

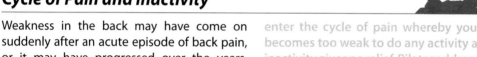

Spinal Stability

If you suffer with back pain, you will be familiar with the ongoing nagging ache and feeling of vulnerability or weakness that it causes in the back. It is this weakness that often leads us to restrict and sometimes actually give up activities that we like to do.

It is a common finding that the more you do, the more the back seems to hurt. Unfortunately, however, it is not the case that the less you do, the less the back hurts. Often, prolonged postures such as standing in line or sitting to watch a film also increase back pain.

Cycle of Pain and Inactivity

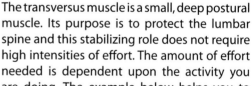

Weakness in the back may have come on suddenly after an acute episode of back pain, or it may have progressed over the years, forcing you to gradually give up more and more of your hobbies over time. If we do not address this weakness with strengthening, you will continue to get weaker and then you enter the cycle of pain whereby your back becomes too weak to do any activity and yet inactivity gives no relief. Pilates addresses this weakness with safe strengthening exercises for the right muscles. These muscles are the corset muscles of the lower abdominals.

The Corset Effect

We have a natural corset of muscles that protect the back; the main stabilizing muscle is the Transversus Abdominal muscle. If you look at the anatomy of this muscle, you will see that it wraps around the lower back and therefore activation of this muscle will give the back a corseting effect, much like a back support does. The purpose of the exercises in this section are primarily to strengthen this muscular corset. Some exercises require the transversus muscle to work maximally and, therefore, you will notice shaking, for example with the plank. Others only require 30 percent effort to protect the back; for example the leg-reach.

The transversus muscle is a small, deep postural muscle. Its purpose is to protect the lumbar spine and this stabilizing role does not require high intensities of effort. The amount of effort needed is dependent upon the activity you are doing. The example below helps you to understand how you can control the effort of tightening your deep abdominals to give your back efficient support:

You need to do some work in the garden but you are restricted due to weakness in the back. To overcome this you tighten your abdominals as hard as you can to give the back as much support

as possible. Rather than feeling better, you actually now will feel more restricted. All your effort is going to tightening the abdominals. You only actually need enough support to save the strain being absorbed by your back, your vulnerable area. To cut the grass with an electric mower, contracting the lower abdominals by 30 percent should be enough to protect the back. If you then begin digging the flower bed when the ground is hard you may feel the back taking the strain; you now need to tighten the abdominals harder to save the back. You find a large root and this needs pulling; now this extra effort is still not enough, so you need to tighten more. The movements that require extra effort require that effort for a shorter time. You may be able to provide that support, you just won't be able to sustain it. It would be like tightening a corset. It may be uncomfortable, but for short bursts will give you the extra support that you need for a quick task.

If you are not very strong in the abdominals, then you may be okay cutting the grass, but you would feel the strain in your back if you were digging or pulling up roots. You need to strengthen first before you move onto more strenuous activities such as these. In this section, the exercises will start at the lower level and if you can control these then you can try to move to the next. If you are trying too hard though, the wrong muscles will work instead. These are called global stabilizers and they do not give the corset effect that we want. You will recognize this by pushing out the abdominals or by tension increasing. As long as you keep to the exercises and functional activities that are within the limits of the strength of your abdominal muscles, that exercise or activity will strengthen, rather than weaken, your back. If, however, you do not activate your abdominals during the exercise or activity, you will not actually be protecting the back at all. It will be like knowing that the back support helps, but forgetting to wear it. It will be clear with the exercises that if you do not activate the abdominal muscles before moving, then you will feel the strain in your back. You will then appreciate the important role of this muscle. Once you understand this role, you will begin applying the principles functionally and will tighten the muscle with daily activities.

Pelvic Stability

If you stand and lift one leg off the floor, does your pelvis tip to the side, lift up or stay level? If your pelvis is stable, the supporting side will remain unchanged by the opposite leg lifting off the floor. Unfortunately, instability is common and one side will be unable to stabilize as the other side moves. This places unnecessary stress through the pelvis. Pelvic instability can be linked with low back pain and may also contribute to any hip, groin, knee or ankle injury. Many sports performers struggle with this section of exercises, despite having good strength of the core muscles.

If the pelvis is not stable, then with every step that you take, you will be placing unnecessary strain through the lower back and pelvis. One of the main muscles responsible for control of pelvic stability is the gluteus medius. This is one of the muscles in the buttocks. It moves the leg from the hip to the side (abduction) and stabilizes the pelvis during walking and other functional activities. Strengthening the gluteus medius muscle requires thought and control, as the movements must be executed correctly to ensure the correct muscle is targeted. The exercises in this section require full concentration, as the movements are subtle and it is not easy to move correctly. If the gluteus medius muscle is weak and the body is not used to recruiting this muscle, then your body will naturally try to cheat. When the correct muscle is isolated you will really feel the benefits.

The best way to understand this section is to think about the activities you do through the day that involve taking one leg off the floor.

When walking, every step you take leaves one leg supporting the body as the other leaves the floor. If you go up a set of stairs, then the moving leg lifts higher and the supporting leg is taking the weight for even longer. With running, even for just a few steps to catch the bus, you are taking your full body weight onto one side. For sports people, supporting weight on one leg can be very relevant; for example, when playing football you are often standing on one leg during each kick of the ball. In martial arts, you need advanced balance and stability to enable you to stand on one leg for a longer period of time as the opposite leg kicks high. If your pelvis cannot remain level when one leg leaves the floor, all these movements will potentially be placing excess strain through the back and pelvis. If you can stabilize the pelvis so that the hips remain level across from one side to the other, you will achieve better control and more efficient movement of the right muscles. You will be more able to isolate the lower limbs to achieve the movements without the back taking the strain. Stabilizing the pelvis can improve individual sports performance, help with balance and improve any discomfort with walking.

Many different factors can affect pelvic stability, including sitting crossed-legged, carrying a child on one hip, being pregnant or having hypermobile joints. Luckily it can be improved with rehabilitation. Working through the exercises in this section will give you a better understanding of balance, control and efficient movement.

Scapular Stability

Look at the posture of those people around you, on the train, in a restaurant or in the office. Shoulders are probably slumped forward, bodies stooped toward the floor and muscles flabby rather than toned. How many people do you know who stand tall, with their shoulders back? Most people look as though the weight of their stresses is pulling their shoulders forward. This is an observation that many of us can relate to, but we do not always understand how it has come to reflect our own bodies! Unfortunately, we are constantly battling against the demands of our society that appear to make a slumped posture easier to achieve than the correct, healthy, upright posture. Once again the repetitive lifestyle that we lead will cause us problems. Generally, in the upper body, our shoulders will be positioned forward and lifted and our upper back will start to show a curve, making us lose height. This posture is now starting at an earlier age and certainly isn't helped by the increase in computer-based activities, especially in young children. We used to see children play outside on their bikes; now the latest computer game console is far more common on a child's Christmas wish list and is rapidly replacing active play.

Joseph Pilates, in his original text 'Return to Life through Contrology,' stated that the human race has not yet adjusted to the demands of modern society. Busy lifestyles tend to be repetitive and often lead to increased stress. We are encouraged to sit more than stand, both at work and to relax. In some respects, lifestyles have become easier; we do not have to hunt for our food like in the days of the caveman, or wash all our clothes and sheets by hand as was normal only seventy years ago. Sofas have modernized; they are soft, offer little support and are often low, but when faced with a choice of this or a hard single chair, which would you choose to relax in? Microwave meals take away the strain of cooking, which is welcomed at the end of a busy day, especially if you have worked late. The problem, though, is that we are not given the opportunity to use our core postural muscles during our everyday activities. If we had to squat to go to the toilet, if we took cushions away from our seating, if we stood to wash our clothes, cooked our meal from scratch and walked from 'a' to 'b' rather than jumping into our cars, then we would be more likely to strengthen and tone our muscles more uniformly than we do with our current fast living or posture-lazy lifestyles. The question is, would returning to a more basic lifestyle and removing our comforts make life more difficult? Our bodies would certainly not then find it easier to slump; we would need good upright posture to deal with everyday activities. Our bodies would have more natural strength, and back pain and tension would also be reduced. With the effects of gravity, it certainly makes more sense to give birth standing than lying flat in a hospital bed! Carrying our shopping in baskets on our heads would mean that weight would be more evenly balanced than our typical means of carrying carrier bags in one hand. If we slept flat on our backs on a hard surface, the muscles shortened through the day would be stretched at night. The dilemma that we face is that what we see as our luxuries are causing our bodies to slump and become weak, yet we would be fools not to use them. Or would we? Replacing our soft sofa with a supportive chair would not be so bad; neither would walking to the grocery store instead of driving. To regain the core strength and posture that we would have had naturally when young, we now need to relearn how this feels and practice applying this new posture functionally for it to become automatic once again! It may sound ridiculous but, unfortunately, it is true. We are spending time and money: relearning what, as children, we did naturally.

So when does it all start to go wrong? If you look at children, they have good posture, they do not slump their shoulders or stoop their backs, because they are constantly moving. It only starts to change when the stresses of society takes over. As soon as this child goes to school, then the body is forced to spend time sitting, often on low, uncomfortable chairs for long periods of the day. It does not help that children carry heavy, awkward rucksacks, often over one shoulder; which will affect posture. Next comes puberty, where we either develop too fast or too slow but either way, slumping the shoulders forward tends to be the natural response of our bodies to hide from the world. Stresses do not disappear as we get older, they simply come from more areas: exams, money, targets at work, family and health. We tend to hold these strains in our shoulders and neck and the feeling of carrying the weight of the world on your shoulders is something most of us can relate to.

Pilates will give you the awareness of the tension you may be holding in your shoulders and neck and will teach you the correct position for your upper body. You will learn how to release this tension, how to stretch the muscles that are often tight and how to strengthen the muscles that are weak. This is an important section for everyone with neck pain, people with tension in their shoulders and neck or anyone with poor posture—so really it is for everyone!

Mobility

Joseph Pilates worked predominantly with dancers in his New York studios. This clientele are naturally flexible as they spend so much time training to improve posture and joint range. Movement is natural to them. When injured, the rehabilitation exercises prescribed need to enable the dancers to return to the full mobility that they had before. The exercises that Joseph taught with Contrology may appear advanced to us but we must remember that the clients he was rehabilitating in his studios were at an advanced level before injury.

When working with the sedentary population, mobility is often a major factor limiting good execution of the original Pilates exercises. We simply spend too much time sitting, and our lives involve too many repetitive movements, as well as not using all of the muscles in our bodies and developing tight muscles. Even people who are involved in sport or gym training are often more concerned with building muscle bulk than improving flexibility. Many sports actually increase muscle imbalance by over-developing certain muscle groups, restricting mobility further; for example, swimmers overwork the muscles at the front of the shoulders and football players overdevelop the muscles at the front of the thigh. In order to improve flexibility, it is important to develop all muscles uniformly, ensuring that no one muscle group is favored.

Joseph Pilates gave the example of the movement of a cat to illustrate how it is natural for animals to stretch thoroughly, both relaxing and stretching each muscle group in turn before rising. If you watch a cat as it goes through the ritual of this stretching routine, it is clear that the cat will not suffer from stiffness and immobility of the joints. This is true of most animals. It is common, however, for we humans to forget this ritual. Our day could accurately be presented as follows:

We wake up, roll out of bed, have a shower, get dressed and get into our car to leave for work. Once at work we sit at our desk, not necessarily moving until lunch. We then move to the staff room to sit and eat. Back to the office for the afternoon, into the car to go home at the end of the day, put some dinner in the microwave, eat dinner, sit to watch TV, go to bed and sleep all curled up.

It is hardly surprising then that our hamstring and hip flexor muscles are tight, as they spend 90 percent of the day in a shortened position. We do not find movement natural, we do not practice it enough. When exercising, it is clear that we need to start at a lower level and build up slowly. Even if you cannot relate to the above example, think about your day. Does it reflect a balance of all your muscles? Or are your daily tasks, however manual, still repetitive? Most of us have repetitive lifestyles and therefore will have tightness in some muscles, causing a lack of natural flexibility. Interestingly, this is not the case in small children, but then they are moving constantly throughout the day. Much like a cat, they wiggle, twist, stretch and bend naturally throughout the course of the day. They certainly do not hold postures for too long.

This section will allow you to work through the exercises that help to improve the mobility of the spine and body. They may appear impossible at present but with perseverance this will improve. It is worth noting, however, that in order to improve mobility it will require you to change your daily habits. At lunchtime, go for a brisk walk rather than sit. Every morning and evening, lie on the floor and do some stretches and mobility exercises. Stop frequently throughout the day to change position and stretch muscles that may be tightening. Lifestyle changes such as these are what the body naturally needs to stay healthy. Pain will begin to improve if you can do this.

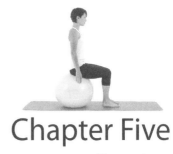

Chapter Five
Understanding & Working through the Assessment Exercises

Spinal Stability

With movements that challenge spinal stability, the focus should be on using the lower abdominal muscles to prevent your back from arching as you move. It is important that the lower abdominals do not release, or you will lose your neutral spine position, causing your pelvis to tip forward. This will cause the back to take the strain. Typically, those with a history of back pain are used to working through pain. Despite knowing that gardening hurts your back, you may continue and simply take a warm bath when you're finished and accept that you will ache the next day. Pilates exercises teach you how to perfect your technique with movements so that you do not experience any strain in your back. You will learn how to move to allow the lower abdominals to stabilize. If you do an exercise and the back hurts, you must stop immediately and assess why. It may be because your technique is wrong and you are arching your back, or you may not have your core muscles protecting your back, either because you have let go or because you are just not strong enough for that particular movement. The purpose of understanding how to alter your technique by using the abdominals to take the strain is that you then begin to accept that you can alter your posture in everyday activities. You will learn to use the abdominals rather than strain your back.

More about the Core Muscles

It is important, before we move on, to understand more about the core muscles. Anatomically, our muscles are in layers and the core muscles are those found in the deepest layer, close to the joints. Due to the deep position of these muscles, it can be difficult to locate or feel them. It is therefore helpful to use imagery to aid our understanding. If we relate to the lower back and abdominals, the postural muscles can be likened to a corset. A corset has a front, back, top and bottom. The front of the corset is represented by the transversus abdominus. This is also known as the "belt buckle muscle" because it runs horizontally across the abdomen below the belly button. The back of the corset is formed by a small group of muscles deep in your back, called the multifidus muscles, that connect your vertebrae. The top of the corset is your diaphragm or "breathing muscle" and the bottom of the corset is made up of the pelvic floor muscles. These muscles together provide an internal support for your spine. The lower back is in danger of being injured if these muscles are weak and not properly trained.

Deep postural muscles act in a different way to the more familiar "global" muscles which are in the outside layer of the body. As many of us have a "lazy" slouching posture, our deep muscles are constantly stretched and this causes them to weaken. As our postural muscles are therefore not developed enough to support our joints, our global muscles take over and work in both a stabilizing and mobilizing role. This causes these outside muscles to overwork and by the end of the day they will feel tired and will ache. Can you relate to a feeling of your head being too heavy for your neck? This is usually a symptom of the deeper neck muscles not stabilizing, with the outside muscles of the neck working to support the weight of the head and move the head as well. As this is more than they are designed to do, the muscles will tire quicker. It is important to train our muscles from the inside out so that they learn to fire in the correct order. The stabilizers will then stabilize, allowing the mobilizers to mobilize. This will lead to more efficient movement, and balance, stability, posture and coordination will all improve. Importantly, there will also be minimal wear and tear on the joints.

30 Percent Rule

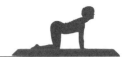

The difference between the effort of the postural muscles compared to the global muscles can be compared to the differences between marathon running and sprinting. If you were to put too much effort into the start of the marathon you will tire and not be able to finish. You need to start at a sensible pace and keep it going. The key to this is endurance. The same is true with the postural muscles; you need ongoing support throughout the whole day. If you waste your energy by trying too hard, then the muscles will tire, give up and you will have no support. To ensure you are not trying too hard, you need to make sure that only the lower abdominal muscle is working and that the correct amount of effort is 30 percent of the full effort you could give. This will effectively target the right muscles to give the right amount of support. You should then be able to maintain this contraction as you continue activities. With all Pilates exercises, you need to maintain this 30 percent effort to ensure that you do not strain the back. It is important to note that there is evidence that faulty activation patterns in the transversus abdominal muscles are associated with a higher risk of recurring back pain. Therefore, in any back rehabilitation program, it is essential to train this muscle.

Locating the Right Muscle

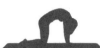

As previously stated, the postural muscles are deep and therefore can be hard to locate. You need to visualize a tight pair of hip-hugger jeans. These jeans will zip up below the belly button and therefore tightening the upper abdominals will not help to master the zip on these jeans. To feel the muscle, place your fingers on your pelvic bones and then move in and down by one inch. If you cough, you will feel the transversus abdominal muscle contract to 100 percent. Now you need to actively tighten this muscle to 30 percent. If you needed 100 percent to do up those jeans, then you couldn't wear them for long! Now, imagine zipping up these hip-hugger jeans by bringing your muscle in beneath your fingers by 30 percent. You should not be holding your breath or holding any tension in the upper tummy or ribcage.

If you find this difficult, you can always try to activate the pelvic floor. This is best thought of as an elevator. At rest, it is on the ground floor. As you try to pull in the pelvic floor it is as though you are trying to stop passing water (please note you must never actually practice this). If you imagine ten floors, as you breathe out, you need to imagine this elevator coming up the floors to the tenth. This will take 100 percent of your effort. You must then gently release the contraction to the fifth floor, then release a bit more to the third floor and this will give you your 30 percent. The most common feedback from clients to this is that it feels as though that couldn't possibly be enough effort to benefit. You wouldn't start the marathon thinking that you aren't putting in enough effort, you would appreciate that you had a long way to run. You need to transfer this thinking to the fact that your postural muscles need to sustain their effort throughout the day.

Neutral Resting Position

This is the position that you will use for all the exercises that begin with you lying on your back.

Lie on your back with your knees bent and your feet flat on the floor, level with your pelvic bones. Your knees should be pelvic distance apart. Find your neutral spine position by flattening your back into the floor, allowing your tailbone to come slightly off the mat. Now do the opposite movement and arch your back so that you could easily put your hands under the curve of your back. Neutral spine is the position halfway between these two extremes. Now relax your upper body so that your ribcage melts into the floor and is not holding tension. Your shoulders should be as close to the floor as possible but be careful not to just lift in the ribcage to achieve this. Your shoulders also need to be away from the ears so that you are not holding tension in the top of your shoulders. Now place your fingers on each pelvic bone found just below your belly button, but to the sides. Move your fingers in and down by 1 inch from these pelvic bones. You are now resting on your transversus abdominal muscle. If you cough or laugh, you will feel the muscle contract.

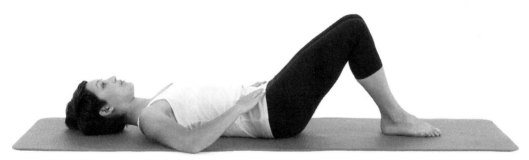

You need to use your abdominal muscles to hold this neutral spine position as you challenge yourself with the movements of the rehabilitation exercises. It is important to engage the correct muscles, the core muscles, to give you this support. The key to working the correct muscle group is to use the correct amount of effort.

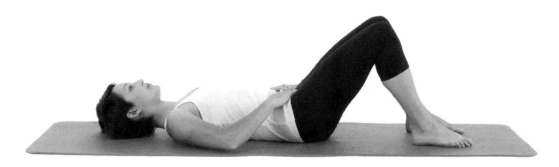

Transversus Holds

To recruit the transversus abdominus muscle, imagine zipping up a tight pair of low-cut trousers. Your fingertips should come slightly closer together as you gently pull in this muscle as you exhale. Avoid tensing the upper abdominals or lifting up the rib cage. The movement is subtle and performed at low intensity.

If you put in 100 percent effort, you may find that your upper abdominals tense too. If you release 70 percent of this effort, you should have the correct 30 percent effort left, with tension only in the lower abdominals. Be careful not to push the abdominals out, but to subtly draw the muscle in. If your muscle is tensing up, then you are trying too hard.

Some people find it difficult to locate the transversus muscle; you may find it easier to target the pelvic floor muscle, which will also give you activity in the deep abdominal muscles. The pelvic floor muscle is tensioned by tightening the muscle that would stop you passing water while going to the toilet. Please note that you should never actually try this as it can disturb bladder flow. You should still remember the 30 percent rule and not overtighten the muscle. The pelvic floor muscle works with the transversus muscle to provide a corset support for the back, the pelvic floor making the bottom of the corset while the transversus forms the front.

Single Tabletop

To Prepare

Start in the neutral resting position.

Engage your lower abdominals with 30 percent effort and exhale to gently float one foot off the floor and up in the air to single table top, as though you are resting this leg on an imaginary table. Imagine that your resting foot is placed on eggshells and, as you lift the opposite foot, you need to think about not breaking these eggshells. This is avoided by not transferring your weight from one foot to the other as you lift the leg. An imaginary glass of water resting below the belly button must not spill as the leg lifts, so keep the pelvis still from right to left.

You should be able to maintain the 30 percent effort in the abdominals to ensure you maintain your neutral spine throughout this movement.

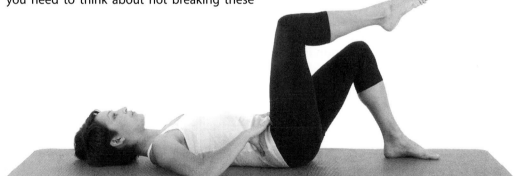

Imprinting

Imprinting is a technique that you can use when performing more advanced movements to give the back extra support. This is when you tilt the pelvis backward to lightly press the back into the floor. This movement protects the spine to prevent you from arching the back or tilting the pelvis forward as you move. If you feel that you need more support with a movement, try this technique and it should help. If your pelvis tips forward, your back is placed under direct strain and you will feel the tension in your lower back. This is how you will know if the exercise level is too advanced for you. You should always be able to maintain neutral or the imprinted position without arching the back as the pelvis tilts forward.

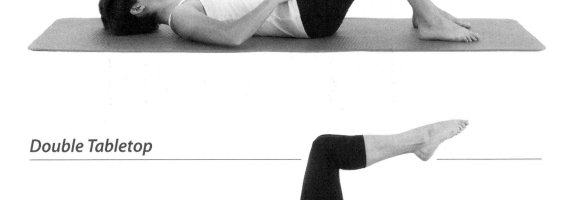

Double Tabletop

Start in the neutral resting position and then float the first leg into single table top.

Make sure you are in neutral and your deep abdominal muscle is engaged. Maintaining either neutral spine or the imprint to give you a little extra support, lift the heel of the second foot and then exhale as you lift the foot off the floor while keeping your lower pelvis still. Your second leg will come into the tabletop position to meet the first leg, using your abdominals to maintain the neutral spine position. This is double tabletop. You may find it easier to scoop the foot in toward the bottom to lift it up as this makes it easier to come into the tabletop position.

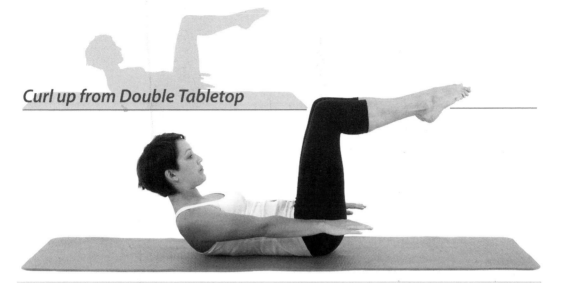

Curl up from Double Tabletop

Start in the double tabletop position.

Exhale as you maintain your double tabletop position and then add the curl-up position lifting from the chest to avoid tensing the neck. Relax the shoulders and neck. Keep a peach distance between your chin and your chest. Your arms are slightly lifted off the floor but your shoulders are pushed down to keep open across the front of the chest.

If you can comfortably control double tabletop without tensing in the upper body and without losing the neutral position of the spine, you can try the following more advanced progressions. Your core abdominal muscles are challenged at the previous levels and you will be able to perform most of the rehabilitation exercises in this section if you can control double tabletop. It is important to understand whether you should stay at single or double tabletop as this will determine which level of the rehabilitation exercises you should be working at. To safely perform the classical Contrology exercises, you need the advanced control and strength challenged by the next two movements.

Double Tabletop Reach

Start in the double tabletop position.

Engage your abdominals and exhale as you slowly reach your legs away from the body to a 45-degree angle without arching your back or letting your pelvis tip forward. As the legs extend away, relax the upper body. The ribs should stay relaxed and the shoulders should not lift. If your abdominals let go, your back will arch and you will feel the strain in your back; you must then bend the knees back to the double tabletop position.

Double Tabletop Reach from Curl Up

Double tabletop reach from curl up is the final progression. Start this from the double tabletop curl-up position. Stretch the legs away, as with the double tabletop reach, but from the curl up.

This level really challenges the upper and lower abdominals, and you will probably feel the muscles shake as you hold the pose.

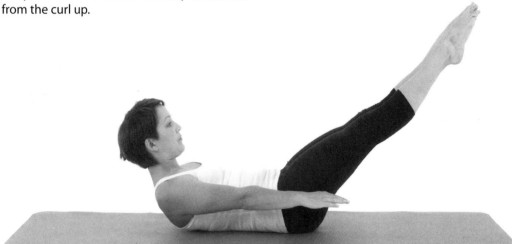

Pelvic Stability

Whether you lie on your back or stand up, if you imagine a carpenter's spirit level across the pelvis from the right to left pelvic bones, you should be able to keep the spirit level as you lift one leg. If you have poor pelvic stability, one side of the pelvis will lift as you move the leg on the opposite side. The lift is subtle and is easy to ignore.

In order for us to make sense of this section, we first need to understand the anatomy of the pelvis. The pelvis can easily be imagined to resemble a basin, as it is a bony ring. It rests on the lower limbs and supports the spine, it is directly attached to the two hip bones and the sacrum (the base of the spine). There are three pelvic joints. The first is the pubic symphysis joint, which is at the front. The second and third are the two sacroiliac joints at the back, which join the pelvic bones to the sacrum. Working together, these joints promote stability during standing, balance, moving, walking and climbing stairs.

The pelvis is subject to constant structural stress because the weight-bearing forces from your two legs is structurally transferred to the central spinal column with every step you take. Because of the repetitive stress of walking, the pelvis is often a source of pain or biomechanical dysfunction. These pelvic joint dysfunctions are often presented as structural or postural imbalances. If the pelvis is not stable during movement, then compensations will occur either above or below. If you consider the position of the pelvis as the base of support for the entire spine, you can understand how pelvic imbalances may refer pain to the lower or middle part of the back, or even the neck or head.

Stability of the pelvis comes from three areas:

1) Bony Structure

The surfaces of the four bones joining together provide what is known to physical therapists as form closure. The stability from joint surfaces provides a form of stability that we have very little control over.

2) Ligament Support

The pelvic ligaments also contribute to form closure. Ligaments join bone to bone. You will find large, strong ligaments in the pelvis. When our posture is bad, the ligaments are either held in a stretched position causing them to weaken, or the stress is increased on the ligaments, causing strain. You cannot directly strengthen the ligaments. Luckily though, we can change our posture. We can compensate for weakness of form closure by improving the strength of the postural muscles around the back, hips and pelvis.

3) Dynamic Muscle Support

The dynamic muscle support is also known as force closure and this is the area that we have the most control over. Pilates is an effective and recognized technique for improving force closure to improve pelvic stability. The exercises in this and the other sections will improve pelvic stability by improving posture to prevent the ligaments stretching and by strengthening the stability muscles.

Through postural bad habits, muscle imbalances develop and the pelvis will be pulled out of line. It is very difficult to successfully rehabilitate instability of the back or pelvis without correcting posture. The most common postural faults are related to the tilt of the pelvis and altered head position. To correct standing and sitting posture, you need to be aware of your own positioning by looking at, and feeling, both the right and the wrong position. If you have shortened muscles in the legs, then the pelvis is pulled into the wrong position and without appropriate lengthening, it will be difficult to alter. Control of the pelvis is necessary to keep the lower spine in correct alignment to prevent low back pain.

The curve of the lower back is controlled by the position of the pelvis. The position that puts minimal strain on the joints and ligaments is the neutral position. If the pelvis tilts forward, the natural lordotic or inward curve of the back is increased. If the pelvis tilts backward, then a flattened back results and the natural curve is lessened. The forward or anterior tilt is the most common postural dysfunction and this posture places extra stress on the ligaments of the spine. This forward tilt is more common in standing and the backward tilt is more common in sitting. In the flat-back posture where the back has lost its natural curve, the muscles and ligaments are stretched and this often leads to back pain.

It is my experience that this is an area that you have to feel to understand, but you do have to concentrate on the movements to achieve quality and control.

The Three Pelvic Positions

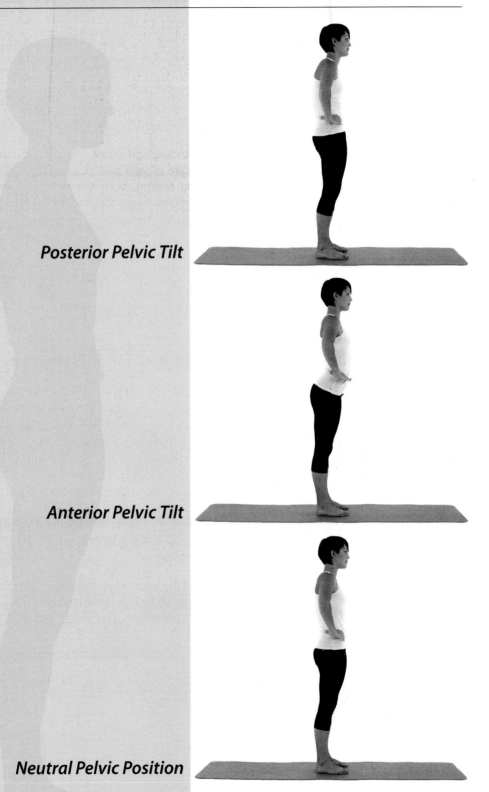

Posterior Pelvic Tilt

Anterior Pelvic Tilt

Neutral Pelvic Position

The Assessment Movements

Single Leg Lift

To Prepare

Start in the neutral resting position.

Engage your lower abdominals to a 30 percent effort and exhale to gently float one foot off the floor to single tabletop. Imagine that your feet are resting on eggshells so that as you lift the foot you do not break the eggshells by transferring the weight to the opposite side. If you had a glass of water resting below the belly button, it should not spill to the sides as the leg floats up. You should be able to lift the leg while keeping steady in the pelvis. Inhale to hold and then gently exhale to lower the leg onto the imaginary eggshells. Repeat on the other side.

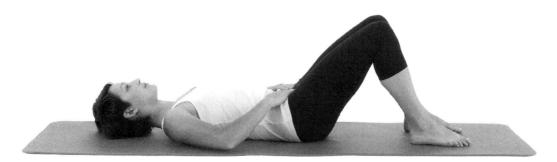

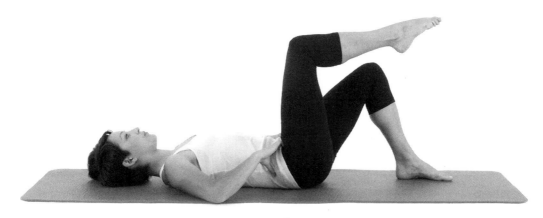

Pelvic Control Drops

Start in the neutral resting position.

Keep your hands on your pelvic bones and be sure that they stay level throughout the movement.

Exhale as you slowly take one knee to the side. Keep the pelvis still throughout the movement. If you are moving the left knee, make sure that the right pelvic bone does not lift. Inhale to bring the knee back and repeat on the other side. Check to see if the movement is more difficult to control on one side. You also need to check that the resting knee stays still, pointing to the ceiling. Imagine a candle resting on this knee and as you take the moving knee to one side, ensure that the resting knee keeps the candle still and doesn't allow the knee to move to the opposite side to counterbalance the movement.

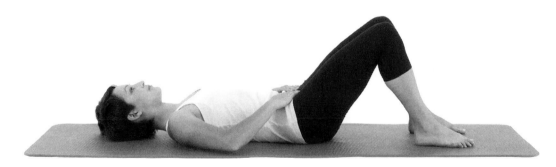

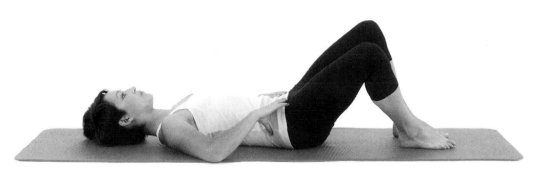

Pelvic Control Lift and Drop

Imagine you have eggshells resting under your feet as you engage your lower abdominals and float one leg into single tabletop. Exhale as you gently take the leg to the side from single tabletop, keeping the knee and foot in line. Be careful not to simply rotate the hip by taking the knee out without the foot. Inhale to bring the leg back. Repeat on the opposite side. As the leg moves to the side, ensure you are keeping the pelvis still; your focus should be on keeping the opposite pelvic bone flat on the floor.

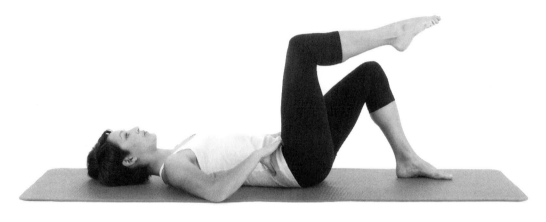

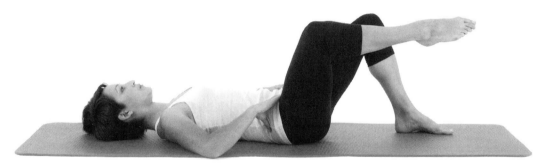

One-Leg Balance

Standing, find your neutral spine by tilting the pelvis both forward then backward and rest halfway between the two.

Place the weight of your body evenly between the heel, big toe and small toe. You should have even weight between the right and left side of the body.

Keep your hands on the pelvic bones as you gently lift the heel on one side and exhale to bring one leg off the floor. Keep the pelvic bones level and the lower abdominals engaged as the leg lifts up. Gently lower the leg and change sides. Begin with a heel lift only and proceed to a leg lift if you are able to control the movement. Try to take the knee forward rather than focusing on hitching the hip up. Begin with small gentle movements and always keep the movement slow.

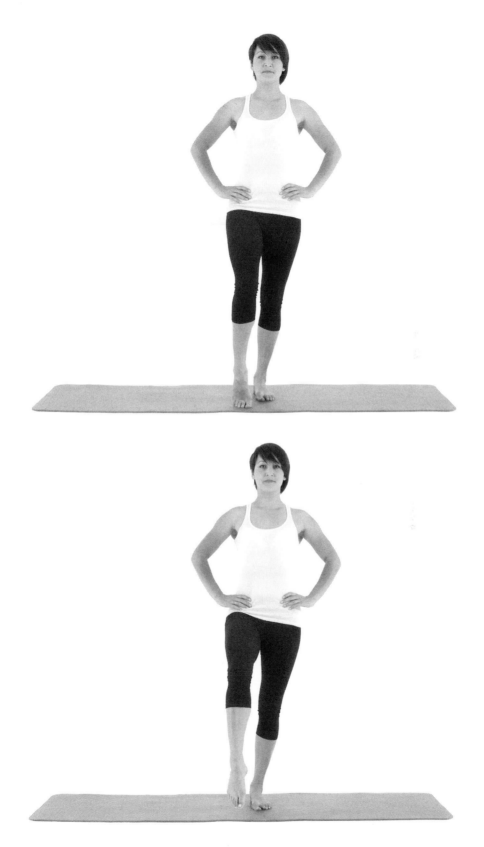

Scapular Stability

Posture

Good posture means that whether you are sitting, standing or lying down, the effects of the force of gravity on our joints, ligaments and muscles is distributed through the body so that there is not excess stress on any one area. Due to the fact that we spend most of our day reaching or leaning forward, we lose this awareness of our alignment and this results in us overstressing structures. We are also often more dominant on one side and this often causes the muscles to develop more on that side. One side may also be more flexible than the other for the same reason.

Most of us have stresses that we tend to hold in our neck and shoulders. This will cause the body to be off balance. It is important to learn to release this tension, as you cannot effectively stabilize through your core if you are holding tension.

When a building is designed, the effects of gravity and weight distribution must be considered. If a building has poor foundations, then the whole structure will be weak and vulnerable. If you have poor posture, then the supporting muscles will be weak and the larger, more powerful muscles will not be able to work as effectively. You will be more susceptible to injury and will suffer more general aches and pains. Performance in sporting or everyday activity will be impaired.

When looking at posture in this section, the focus is on the upper body. As mentioned previously, in a resting position, due to so much of our activity being carried out in front of us, our shoulders are often in a forward position, this will causing our heads to poke forward and then our upper backs become rounded. At its extreme, in a sitting position, the lower back will also become rounded. Unfortunately, this is not uncommon. In this forward position, the weight of the head is not balanced over the spine and therefore the deep postural muscles and ligaments will be stretched. When stretched, they will become weak and their sensitivity to activate will lessen. The neck will then not have the support that it needs, holding the head will become a strain and tension will increase. Trying to correct this will not be easy, as the stabilizing muscles and ligaments will weaken. You will lose the subconscious reaction to correct posture. It all sounds very bad, but luckily, Pilates comes to the rescue! Pilates will teach you how it feels to relax your upper body and will increase your awareness of good posture. You will then be ready to challenge this posture with movement. It is important though, that with movement we do not fall straight back into our old slouching posture, which is exactly what the body will want to do.

So what is good posture?

We have already said that it is when the forces of gravity are evenly distributed through the joints. We also know that the head should be directly above the neck. It is very difficult though to get the upper body posture right if we do not have the pelvis in the right position. So first we need to find our neutral spine and then we'll move up the body to the top of the head. We'll assess upper body posture in sitting as this is functional. It is where we spend most of the day and it is the position that tends to lead us into trouble in the first place. We need to be able to then transfer our new knowledge of good posture into function. It therefore makes sense to do these exercises in functional positions as well as lying down.

In a sitting position, we should have our knees bent and our hips and knees should be at 90 degrees. The weight through our feet should be even on the right and the left, without the feet being arched or flattened.

Aligning the pelvis: Hold the pelvis so that your thumbs are at the back and your fingers are at the front. Imagine you are holding a bucket of water. First tip the pelvis forward, then backward; halfway between these two extremes is neutral. Stay in this position and you will already be a little taller.

Think about the shoulders. Position the shoulders so that they are in line with the spine. Try not to force them back as this will cause the ribs to flare. Imagine someone is pushing down on your shoulders so that they do not lift up. The action is more of a gentle down and back softening of the shoulder blades. If you think of a string pulling the bottom corners of the shoulder blades together this will have the same effect.

The head needs to be lifted. Imagine a helium balloon lifting the back of the head. Your chin will tuck in and this will give you a subtle double chin. You do not want your head and chin poking forward. The head should be directly floating above the shoulders.

You are now aligned correctly. You will have grown, but you will probably feel that this position is causing effort in muscles you were unaware of. You will be unable to hold this position for long. This simply proves the weakness of the stabilizing muscles. You need to try to practice this position as often as you can to address this weakness and you will soon find the posture easier.

With the exercises in this section, it is vital that you maintain this posture throughout. This may mean keeping to a lower level. The aim is to challenge the posture, but not lose it. As soon as it is lost, you will no longer be benefiting and you will not improve your posture. It is extremely beneficial to do these exercises in front of a mirror. You will need as much feedback as possible at first to know that you are doing the movements correctly. You will not be able to rely on feeling that you have not lifted the shoulders, you will need to watch and feel. This section is not easy to master, but you will improve with practice.

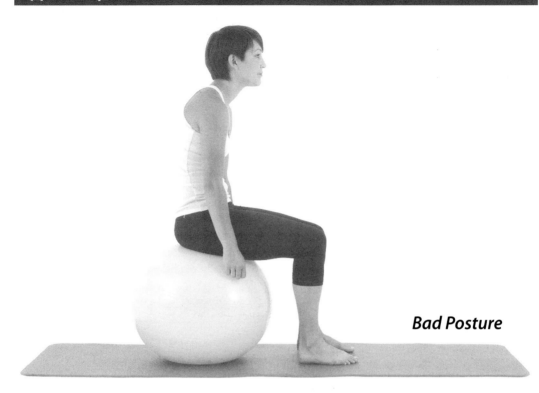

Bad Posture

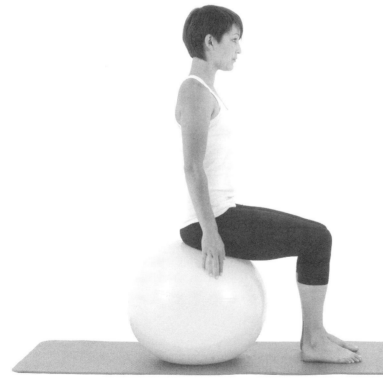

Good Posture

Mobility

Begin this section by answering the following questions:

- Can you touch your toes?
- If you side bend, can you reach past your knees on both sides?
- Can you easily twist your body when driving to see behind you?
- Can you move your head to see someone sitting next to you without needing to twist your body?
- Can you reach your arm around your back to touch the bottom of your shoulder blades?

Did you answer yes to all or most of the above? If so then you have naturally good flexibility. If you cannot touch your toes, it could be that your back or hamstrings are tight. If you cannot side bend, then the quadratus lumborum muscle (found in your lower back) may be restricting your movement. To be able to rotate your body, your thoracic spine (or mid back) should be free to move; if not, then you will twist your hips too, which places an unnatural strain on the pelvis. If you cannot look over your shoulder with just neck movement, then you have shortened muscles in the neck. You are probably holding tension in the neck and typically this will have been caused by poor posture.

The position in which we eat, sleep, stand, sit, work and move influences our posture. Poor posture, or sedentary or repetitive lifestyles, can cause your spine to be compressed and this places enormous amounts of stress on surrounding muscular and connective tissues. If the muscles are tight, then there will be more stress to the tendons and ligaments and there will be a higher risk of injury.

What Is Flexibility?

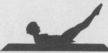

Flexibility is the range of movement of a joint, or series of joints, e.g. the joints of the lumbar or thoracic spine. If the joints do not have the full range of movement, then they will be susceptible to injury with certain activities, particularly active sports participation. Individuals with more range of movement have fewer limitations in their ability to live life. Tightness will impede normal movement and muscles weaken when movement is limited.

It is important to note that flexibility is joint specific. This means that you could have good movement in one joint while being stiff in another. For example, you may easily be able to reach behind the back due to good shoulder flexibility but may be tight in your back and hips, making touching your toes seem impossible.

Flexibility and Posture

As our bodies tend to adopt altered positions or postures, certain muscles will be held in a shortened position. True flexibility requires good length of your muscles. Muscles become tight when they are not stretched. If you have a repetitive lifestyle without enough varied movement in your daily routine, then certain muscles will never get the stretch that they need to maintain flexibility. There are certain muscles that are prone to shortening, directly due to our posture. The muscles that get tight include those in the back of the thigh, the front of the hips, the buttocks, the calf, the inside thigh and the back. Tightness in these muscles can affect posture and is often a source of spinal pain. An example is that if the hamstrings are tight, they may pull the pelvis into a posterior tilt position that stretches the ligaments, causing low back pain.

Mechanical Back Pain

Those of us who have suffered an episode of low back pain will agree that the pain can be excruciating and debilitating. You go to your local GP clinic, looking for an answer, simply to be told "you have back pain." You want a more accurate diagnosis to explain the pain that you are in. The truth is that many incidences of low back pain can be covered under the umbrella term "mechanical low back pain." This basically means that the pain is coming from the moving parts of the back and that the back is simply not moving as it should. There is not a more accurate diagnosis and blood tests, X-rays and MRI scans will all come back clear. Mechanical low back pain does not mean there isn't a real diagnosis, it is a diagnosis and it is recognized as potentially being severe and restricting to a normal lifestyle, particularly by anyone who has experienced similar problems. Think about the mechanics of an engine: if you do not look after the engine as you should it will seize up and stop working. You would not be surprised if you haven't changed the oil, serviced the car regularly and used the engine, yet we abuse our bodies with poor posture, repetitive lifestyles and general immobility and are surprised when we have pain. The answer to mechanical back pain is not just to move, but to move as the back was designed to move. This means correcting posture to ensure you are upright and balanced. You also need to regularly change position, avoiding sustained postures so that you are not putting too much stress on certain muscles, causing them to shorten. Stretching does not have to mean lying on the floor holding a stretch. Simply changing position will give muscles a stretch. Lengthening muscles will not be a quick fix. Be prepared for it to take weeks, usually months, of stretching to mobilize the spine and soft tissues. But it does work. If you are committed, you will gain relief from pain, find general movement much easier and your incidence of injury should be reduced.

The exercises in this section will focus on improving shoulder, back and hip mobility. The important thing to note is not only how much movement you have, but also where you are moving from. For example, you may be able to twist your body to look to one side, but are you moving from your mid back or are you twisting at the pelvis? Also be aware of any differences between one side of the body and the other. This could be related to your lifestyle. For example, if you are able to twist one way easier than the other, could this be because you watch the TV at an angle with your body twisted? Or do you twist to type at work? By changing bad habits during your everyday activities, your mobility could improve dramatically.

It is always important to remember that it is far better to do a lower level well than cheat to achieve a higher level. Concentrate on the teaching points and be prepared for the improvements in this section to take a while to have an effect.

The Assessment Movements

Thoracic Rotation

To Prepare

Sit with your arms across your chest and your legs extended in front of you (if this is uncomfortable, bend your knees or sit on a foam block). Imagine your pelvic bones are spotlights and they must stay pointing forward throughout the movement.

The Rotation

Keep your head and breastbone aligned as you exhale to rotate the upper body in one direction. Inhale to hold and then exhale to return. Repeat to the other side.

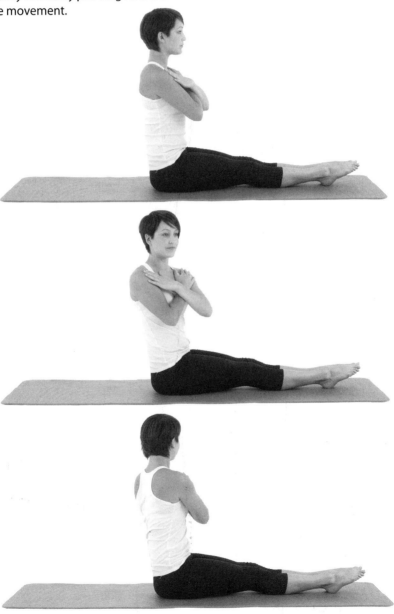

C-Curve Position

To Prepare

Sit with your knees bent and your feet flat on the floor. Hold your arms up in front of you so that they are level with your shoulders. Relax your shoulders. Tuck your chin into your chest.

Exhale as you tuck your tailbone under and roll the pelvis backward. Continue to roll the pelvis back as you reach the arms forward. Your lower back should begin to press into the floor as your upper body reaches forward making a 'C' position of the spine.

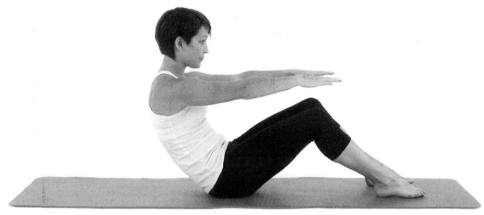

Hamstring Stretch

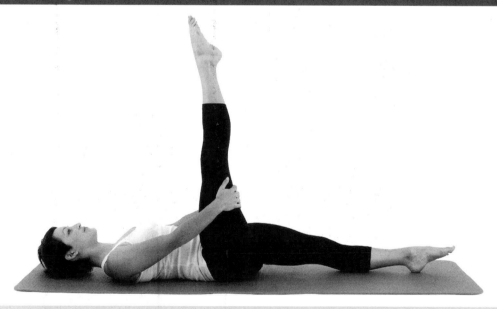

Lying on your back with one leg straight on the floor, bring the other leg up in the air and hold the leg toward you, supporting the leg behind the thigh. To feel the stretch in the back of the thigh, slowly straighten the leg.

Keep your foot relaxed and hold the stretch for 30 seconds. After each 10 seconds, use the exhalation to gently stretch the leg a little bit more without straining the muscle. Repeat on the other side.

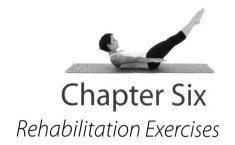

Chapter Six
Rehabilitation Exercises

Leg Reach

The leg reach series strengthens the lower abdominals and tones the front of the legs.

Teaching Points

The further you reach the leg away from the body, the more control you need from your core to maintain a neutral spine. If you feel your back arching, you must stop and return the leg so that you do not strain the back.

This movement prepares you for the single leg stretch exercise in the Contrology section.

To Prepare

Start in the resting position. Imagine your feet are resting on eggshells.

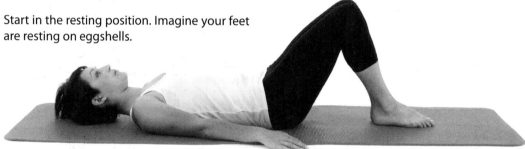

Gently float one leg off the floor without lifting the opposite pelvic bone and exhale to reach the leg away without arching the back. Inhale to return. Repeat on the other side. Continue for 8 reaches on each side.

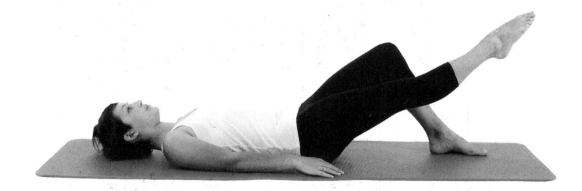

Double Tabletop Leg Reach

If you can control double tabletop without straining the back, begin this progression from double tabletop and then reach one leg away from here. You may find that the back arches before you actually reach fully so be aware as to how far you can safely reach.

Curl Up Double Tabletop Reach

This will challenge the upper abdominals as well as the core. Lift from the chest to avoid tensing the neck.

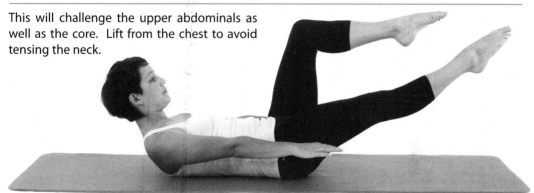

Opposite Arm Reach

This will challenge the scapular stability and increase the challenge to the core by using longer levers. As the arm reaches overhead, do not lift the ribcage or allow the shoulders to travel toward the ears. This also challenges coordination!

You can add the arms to the legs from single leg reach or from double tabletop.

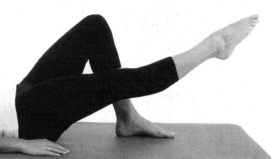

Leg Lowers

This exercise challenges both the upper and lower abdominals. It also stretches the hamstrings.

Teaching Points

With this movement be sure to maintain a neutral spine as the leg lowers. This requires strength and control of the abdominals.

Keep the leg straight as it lifts back up toward the ceiling so that you feel a stretch in the hamstring muscle.

To Prepare

Start in the resting position and reach one leg up in the air to a 90-degree angle, maintaining a neutral spine.

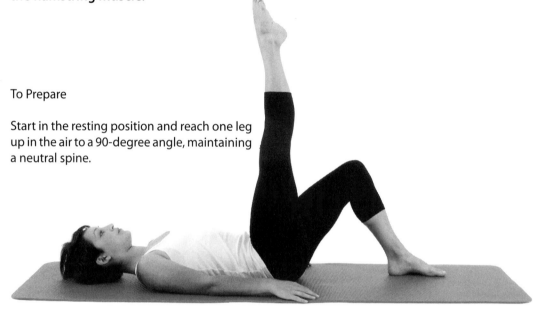

The Leg Lower

Exhale to gently lower the leg down toward the floor, keeping your pelvis in neutral. Do not allow your back to arch. Inhale to hold and then exhale to float the leg back up to the ceiling without allowing the knee to bend.

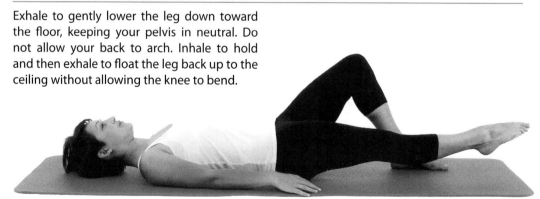

From Double Tabletop

This is a harder exercise because you need more abdominal control to maintain the neutral spine with the resting leg in the tabletop position. The movement is the same as before.

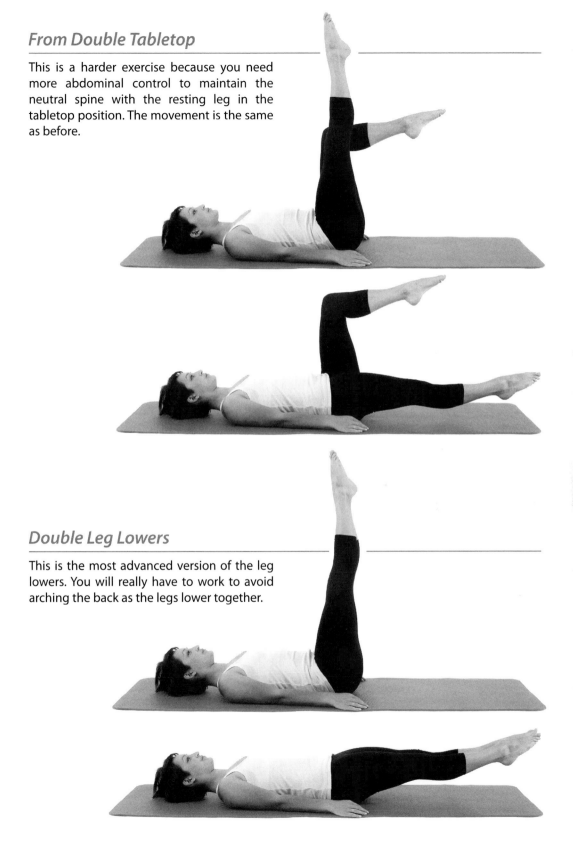

Double Leg Lowers

This is the most advanced version of the leg lowers. You will really have to work to avoid arching the back as the legs lower together.

The Bicycle

This exercise challenges the abdominals and will strengthen the front of the legs.

Teaching Points

The bicycle movement should be a reciprocal movement; the challenge is to reach each leg away from the body in a continuing flowing movement without allowing the pelvis to tip forward.

You must be careful not to tense the upper body with this movement.

To Prepare

Start in the resting position and then reach one leg out, keeping it on the floor. Reach the other leg up into the air at 90 degrees.

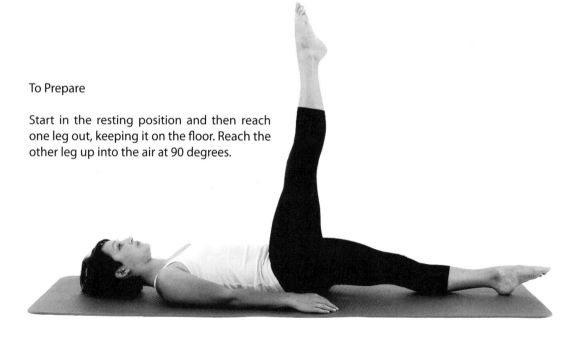

1. Exhale to bring the resting leg off the floor and begin to scoop the leg into the body. The second leg begins to lower to the floor.

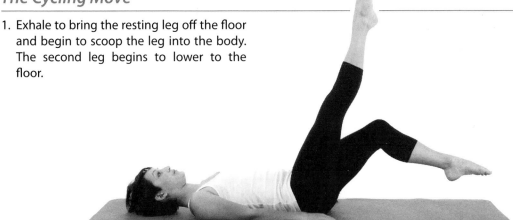

2. Continue to exhale as the lowering leg comes down further toward the floor and the scooping leg comes in toward the chest.

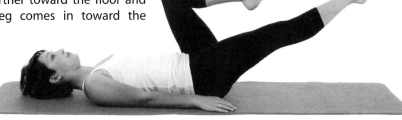

3. Now scoop the lowering leg in toward the body and reach the scooped leg away to begin lowering.

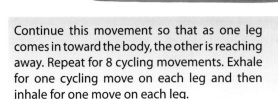

Continue this movement so that as one leg comes in toward the body, the other is reaching away. Repeat for 8 cycling movements. Exhale for one cycling move on each leg and then inhale for one move on each leg.

The movement can be advanced by starting in and sustaining a curl-up position or by changing the direction of the cycling as though you are pedaling backward for 8 more cycles.

Curl Up

This exercise works the abdominal wall. The rectus abdominal muscle is the six-pack muscle at the front of the abdominals. The curl up uses the transversus abdominal muscle to wrap around the back to stabilize the spine while the upper abdominals bring the upper body off the floor.

Teaching Points

The most common mistake with a curl up is to come up too high and have strain in the back. As long as the deep abdominal muscle is contracted, the back is supported. It is important to move from the upper body, keeping the body still below the rib cage.

It is also common to have strain in the neck with this exercise. You must let the weight of the head relax into your hands as you come up.

Starting with your knees bent, you can vary the movement by beginning with straight legs or by adding a leg lift to each curl up.

If you can control the curl up then you can add it to many of the exercises in this section to increase the challenge on spinal stability and strength.

To Prepare

Bend your knees so that your feet are flat on the floor. Place your hands behind your head and let the weight of your head relax into your hands. Keep your elbows wide so that you are not holding tension in your upper body. Engage your lower abdominals to protect your back.

The Curl Up

Exhale to curl your upper body up from the chest and work your upper abdominals. Inhale to lower. Repeat 8 times.

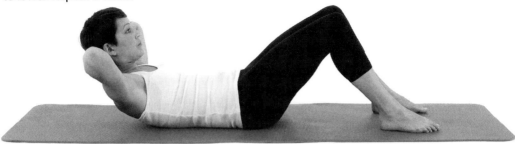

Adding Single Leg Lift

As you curl up, you can increase the challenge on the lower abdominals by adding a single leg lift. Keep still while moving from right to left and be sure that the pelvis does not tip to the sides or tilt forward as you lift a leg.

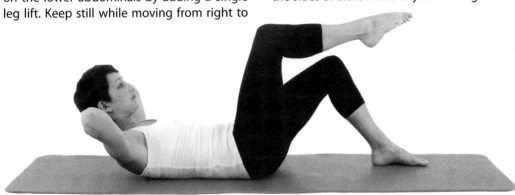

From Double Tabletop

Maintaining a double tabletop position as you curl is hard and makes the curl up very effective for challenging both the lower and upper abdominals. Correct technique is crucial for achieving the most from this exercise. Do not swing up or tense the upper body. Keep the pelvis still throughout.

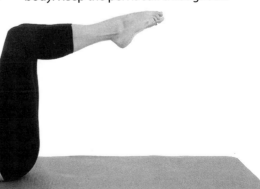

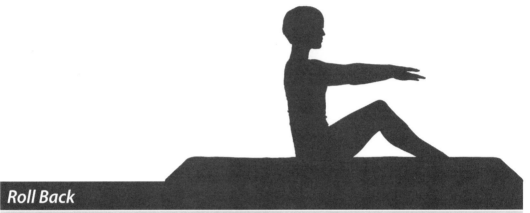

Roll Back

This exercise mobilizes and opens the spine and strengthens the deep abdominal muscles.

It is an important exercise for facilitating segmental motor control and it demonstrates the level of your ability in controlling your spinal movement.

Good execution of this movement requires mobility of the spine, especially at the lumbar region. You also need good abdominal strength to keep the movement controlled.

Teaching Points

This exercise should be started with bent knees and then advanced to straight legs.

You can do the movement with your arms down, rather than up at shoulder height, if they feel too heavy.

It is important with this exercise that you do not initiate movement from your upper back. Initially you must roll from the pelvis, creating movement in your lower back. It may help to place your hands in the small of your back as you roll back so that you know you are initiating the movement from the right place. Once you know that you are doing the movement correctly you can bring your arms back in front of you.

The roll back is a preparatory exercise for the roll up.

The Roll Back

To Prepare

Bend your knees, keeping your feet flat on the floor. Engage your abdominal muscles and exhale as you tuck your tailbone under.

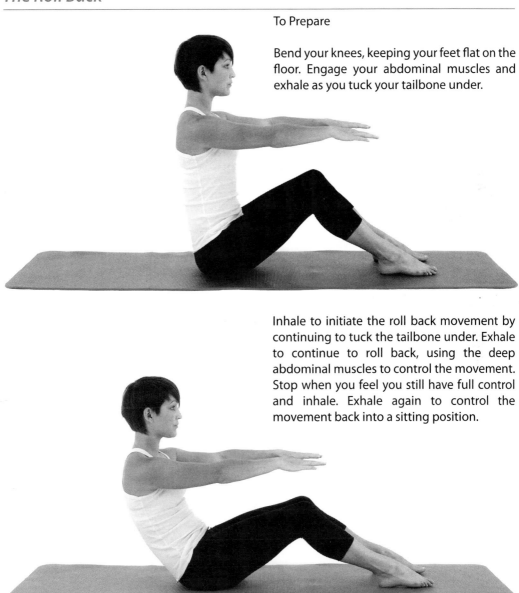

Inhale to initiate the roll back movement by continuing to tuck the tailbone under. Exhale to continue to roll back, using the deep abdominal muscles to control the movement. Stop when you feel you still have full control and inhale. Exhale again to control the movement back into a sitting position.

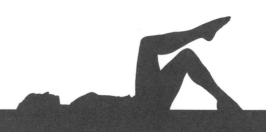

Bent Knee Scissors

This exercise challenges reciprocal movement of the legs. Stability during the movement of the legs should transfer to functional movements such as walking or running.

Teaching Points

With this exercise you must use your deep abdominal muscle to act like a corset to protect the spine and ensure you do not lose neutral, as one leg comes into a single leg lift. You then change legs, either changing in the air or keeping one foot lightly pressed on the floor.

Imagine that your feet are resting on eggshells to challenge pelvic stability. Be careful not lift in the pelvis as you change feet. Initially, keep your hands either side of the pelvic bones and make sure they stay level throughout the movement.

When you know that you are safe in your lower back and that your abdominals are supporting you, you can think about your shoulders. As you progress, be sure that you do not tense in the upper body.

Begin with the single leg lift to correct technique and then move into the bent knee scissors. The progression is the straight leg scissor in the Contrology exercises.

To Prepare

Start in the resting position, imagining eggshells resting under the feet.

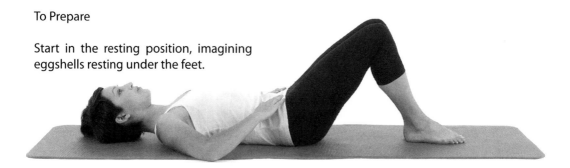

The Scissor Movement

1. Inhale to gently float one leg off the floor, to single tabletop, keeping your deep abdominals activated to protect the back.

2. Exhale to deepen the abdominal contraction and bring your other foot off the floor, heel first, as you bring the first foot down.

3. Repeat for 8 changes.

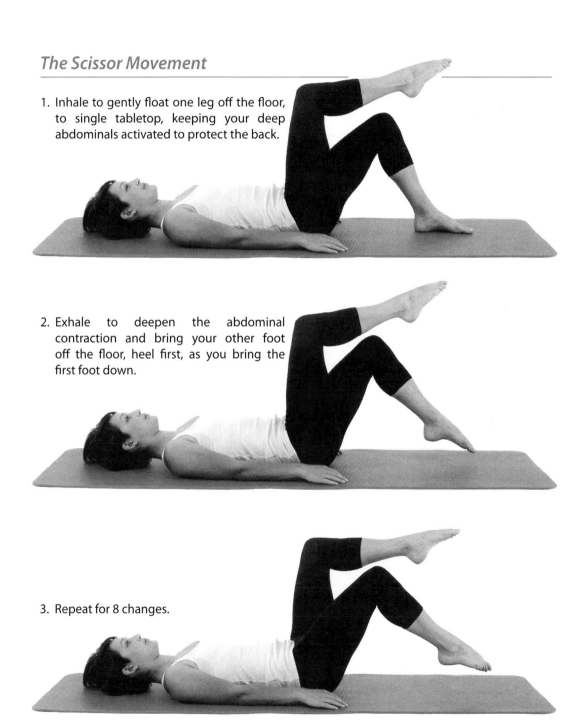

Pelvic Rolls

This exercise uses the abdominal muscles to control the movement of the pelvis rolling from one side to the other.

At the lower level this is a great exercise for back pain. It gently encourages the back to move.

Teaching Points

It is important to use your shoulder blades to anchor the upper body with this movement. Be careful not to allow your upper body to roll too, or you will not be able to come back safely using the abdominals.

Relax the legs throughout this movement. Do not allow the knees to pull you back.

You can relax your neck and let the head move in the opposite direction to of your legs.

To Prepare

Start in the resting position, but have your knees and feet together. Take your arms slightly wider apart and sink your shoulder blades into the floor.

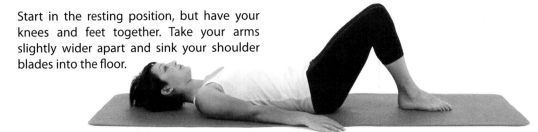

The Pelvic Roll

1. Engage your lower abdominal muscle and inhale to allow your knees to roll over to one side. Make sure to keep both shoulder blades anchored to the floor. Exhale to use your abdominals to control the move back to the center.

2. Continue now with the same movement on the opposite side. Perform 8 rolls in each direction.

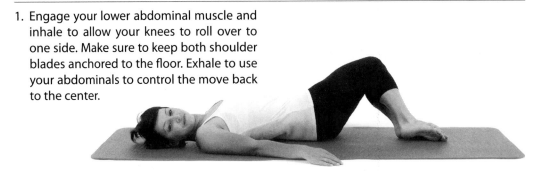

Double Tabletop Pelvic Roll

This is a harder version, as you are required to maintain a neutral spine with double tabletop and move from there. Note that you will not have as much movement from this position as you roll.

Straight Leg Pelvic Roll

To improve hamstring length, you can take this exercise further by keeping both legs straight. This increases the load on the abdominals, making the movement much harder on the core.

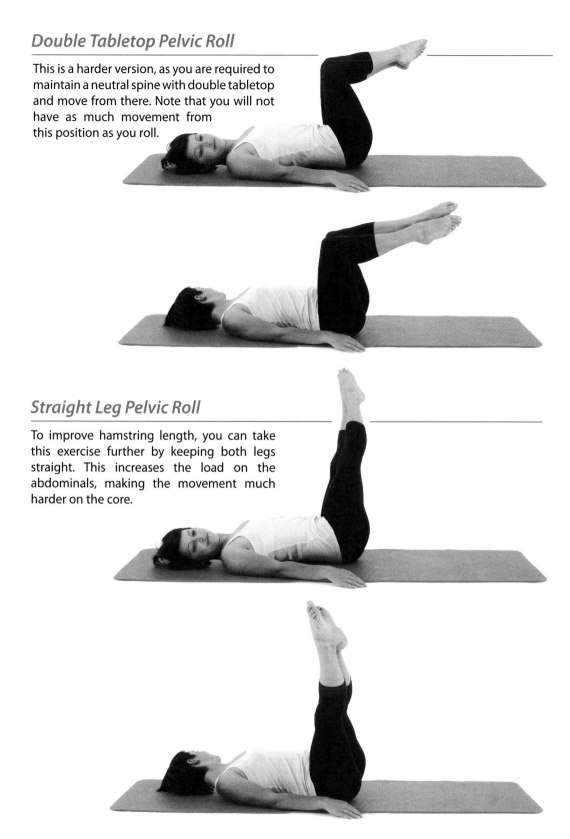

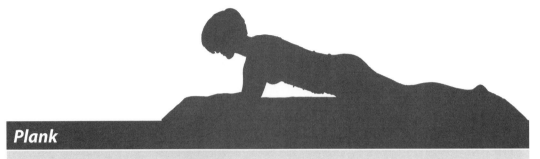

Plank

The plank is a challenging exercise that develops core strength and spinal stability.

Good control and technique of the plank requires strength and stability of the arms, gluteus muscles (the buttocks!) and legs.

The plank traditionally comes from the yoga plank pose position. It is becoming increasingly used within the Pilates matwork program to strengthen the core.

Teaching Points

Always start from the modified plank, resting on your knees and then advance to the full plank onto your toes.

You will probably feel the abdominal muscles shake with the plank. This is because you are working the deep abdominals very hard and they are not used to working in this way. The shaking is just the exertion of this muscle.

The twist and full leg pull are movements that can be tried if the plank can be safely performed at the advanced level.

To Prepare

On your front, rest on your forearms, keeping your shoulders drawn down and away from the ears. Now tuck the tailbone under and peel the pubic bone away from the floor, keeping a straight back and neutral spine.

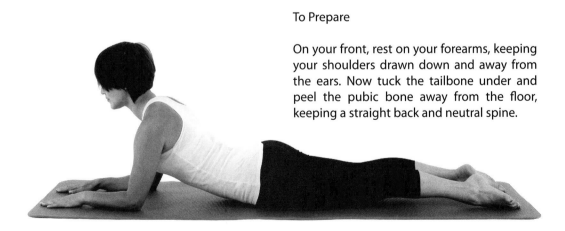

The Modified Plank

Exhale as you continue to peel away from the floor so that the front of your hips come away from the floor and you are resting on your knees. Now hold this position for 10 to 60 seconds.

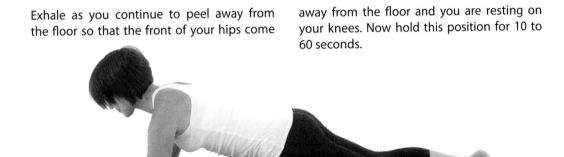

The Full Plank

Continue to peel away, lifting the knees, straightening the legs and holding the position with your feet supporting you.

Hold the plank for 10 to 60 seconds. Keep breathing. Keep your tailbone tucked under to support your back.

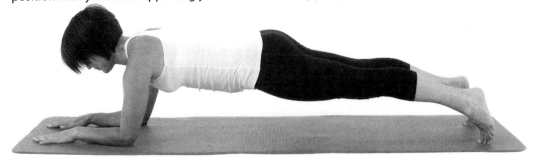

The twist requires excellent core control, good arm strength and scapular control.

Teaching Points

Keep your body aligned throughout the movement without allowing the body to roll either forward or back.

This advanced exercise should only be attempted if you can control the side bend and full plank.

To Prepare

Bend your knees and sit on the outside of your left hip and leg. Place your right foot flat on the floor in front of your left ankle. Place your left hand on the floor and reach your right arm to the side.

Inhale, lifting up through your spine, then exhale completely.

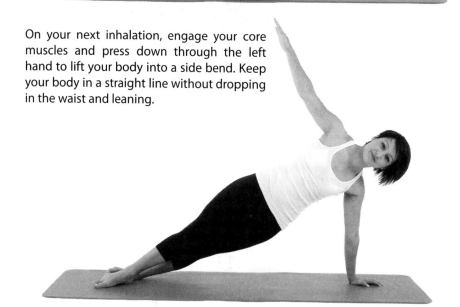

On your next inhalation, engage your core muscles and press down through the left hand to lift your body into a side bend. Keep your body in a straight line without dropping in the waist and leaning.

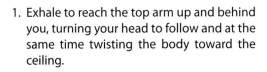

The Twist

1. Exhale to reach the top arm up and behind you, turning your head to follow and at the same time twisting the body toward the ceiling.

2. Inhale to hold and then exhale to bring the arm back down toward the floor so that your body is coming forward, facing the ground.

3. Repeat up to 5 times and then relax.

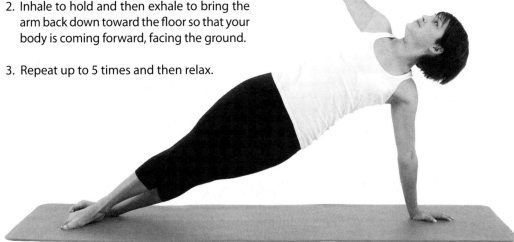

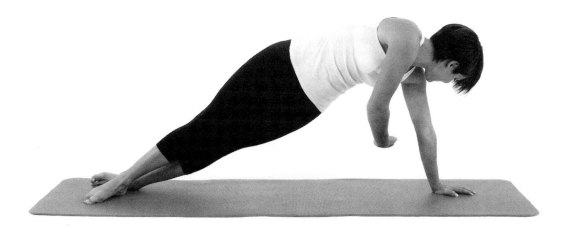

Clam Series

The clam series targets the muscles that control pelvic stability, namely the gluteus medius muscle. It is the best exercise for increasing awareness of this stabilizing muscle that we often do not even know exists!

Improving pelvic stability will also improve hip mobility and will tone the hip and thigh muscles.

Teaching Points

The focus is on grounding the pelvis and spiraling from the inner thigh to raise the knee. Taking the knee away from the hip rather than focusing on the lift.

The clam is an important exercise to master before advancing to the side kick series.

To Prepare

Lie on your side with your knees bent. Your shoulders and hips should be stacked directly one on top of the other and your feet should be in line with your hips. Keep your top arm in front for support. Lengthen away from the waist, so that you are not collapsing into the floor. Maintain a neutral pelvis position.

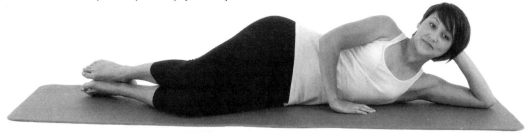

The Standard Clam

Engage your deep abdominal muscle, exhale and bring the top knee up and away from the hip, keeping the feet together. Maintain the neutral pelvic position. Don't roll back or lift from the waist. Inhale to return. Repeat 10 times.

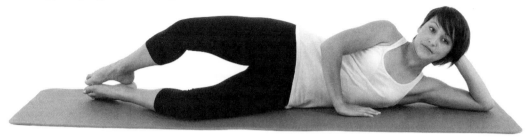

The Elevated Clam

Lift both feet off the floor together keeping your pelvis still. Engage your deep abdominal muscle, exhale and bring the top knee up and away from the hip, keeping the feet together. Maintain the neutral pelvic position. Don't roll back or lift from the waist. Inhale to return. Repeat 10 times.

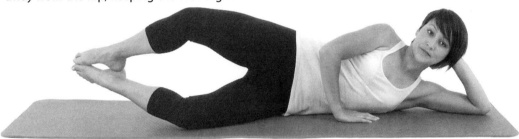

The Reach Away Clam

Engaging your deep abdominal muscle, inhale and bring the top knee up and away from the hip, keeping the feet together. With the knee still, exhale and reach the top leg away from the body. Bring the feet back together and inhale, lowering the top knee. Continue, repeating 10 times.

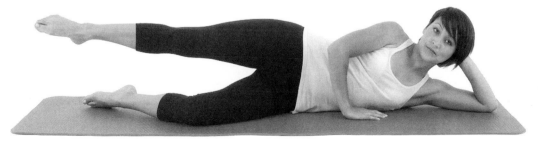

This series of exercises works the lateral rotators of the hips. These muscles are responsible for pelvic stability, and weakness of these muscles often leads to low back pain.

This exercise will also tone the inner and outer thigh, the buttocks, the hips and the front of the legs.

Teaching Points

It is important to get the preparatory position right before you can successfully do the kicking movements. The core muscles will be challenged to maintain this position as you isolate movement to the hip joint. You will need to start with a smaller range of movement and then make the movements bigger and quicker as you increase stability.

To make this exercise easier, bend the supporting leg. If it is uncomfortable on your neck, place a three-inch pillow under your head instead of the bent arm.

You can vary this exercise by doing the same series in a standing position. You just need to be sure you get the right starting position. You will work the gluteus muscle in both the supporting and moving leg. Performing this movement while standing also requires good balance.

Prepare for this series with the clam series. As you strengthen these muscles you will be able to master the more advanced side kick in kneeling.

To Prepare

Lie on your side with your legs straight and your underneath arm supporting your head. Your shoulders and hips should be stacked directly under one another and in a straight line. Find your neutral spine position to ensure that you are not arching or flattening your back. Lengthen away your top hip now from the waist so that you are not collapsing onto the floor (see gap under waist). The top arm should be in front assisting with balance. The bottom leg will anchor the body. You can rotate the top leg from the hip so that the toes point to the ceiling.

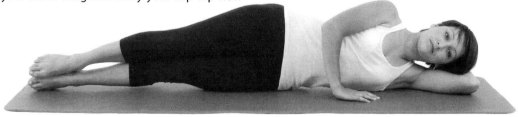

Lifting Kicks

1. Exhale to reach the top leg away from the body and float the leg up to hip height. Inhale to hold.

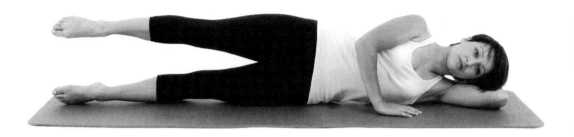

2. Exhale to lift the leg higher maintaining the neutral position of the spine and not lifting in the hip. Inhale to lower the leg to hip height again. Repeat as you exhale again. Continue for 8 lifts.

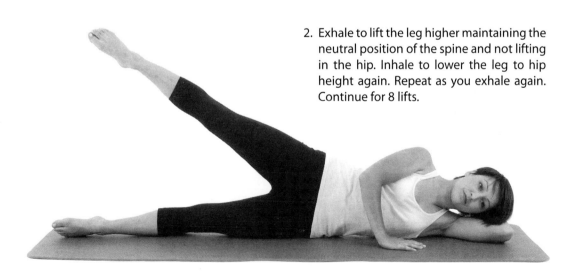

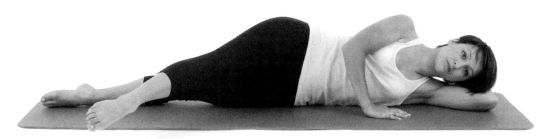

Forward Kicks

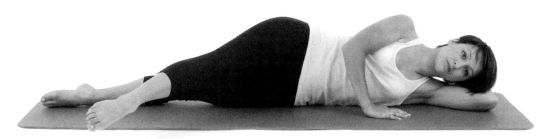

1. Exhale to reach the top leg away from the body and float the leg up to hip height.

2. Inhale to glide the leg forward and then exhale to move the leg backward, keeping the pelvis in neutral. You must be careful not to let the pelvis tip backward, as the leg comes forward, or the pelvis tip forward as the leg moves backward. Continue for 8 kicks.

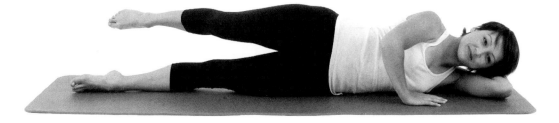

Lift & Circle

1. Exhale to reach the top leg away from the body and float the leg up to hip height. Inhale to hold.

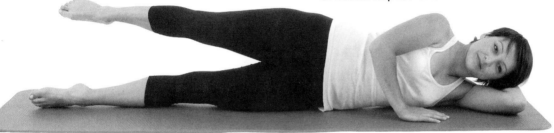

2. Exhale to circle the leg from the hip in a clockwise direction. Repeat. Now inhale to continue with another 2 circles in the same direction. Repeat for 8 circles.

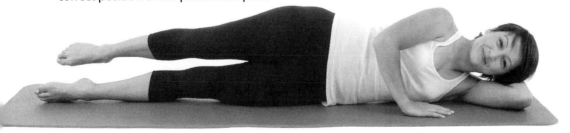

3. Continue with the above movements but in an counterclockwise direction for 8 circles. Make sure that you do not lose the correct position of the pelvis and spine.

Side Cycling

This advanced pelvic stability exercise will tone all the hip and thigh muscles.

This exercise is a real challenge to the abductor muscle group, as abduction of the hip is maintained while a cycling motion is added. The gluteus medius muscle will work throughout and this is the muscle you will feel burn!

Teaching Points

The pelvis must be kept still as movement is isolated to the hip joint.

This is the most advanced pelvic stability exercise of the side lying pelvic rehabilitation exercises. The Contrology shoulder bridge and side kick in kneeling are the exercises you will progress to when you have mastered the side cycling.

To Prepare

Lie on your side with your legs slightly bent and your underneath arm supporting your head. Your shoulders and hips should be stacked directly under one another and in a straight line. Find your neutral spine position to ensure that you are not arching or flattening your back. Lengthen away your top hip from the waist so that you are not collapsing onto the floor. The top arm should be in front, assisting with balance. Straighten your top leg and lift the leg off the floor.

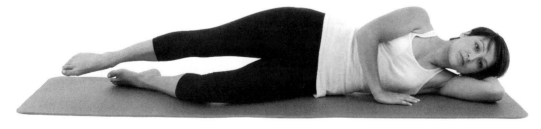

Side Cycling

1. Inhale to bring your foot in toward your buttocks.

2. Now flex the hip so that your knee comes toward your chest, maintaining a neutral spine.

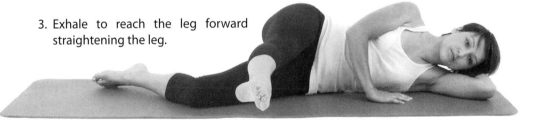

3. Exhale to reach the leg forward straightening the leg.

4. Continue to exhale as you bring the straight leg back in line with the body.

Repeat this movement 8 times.

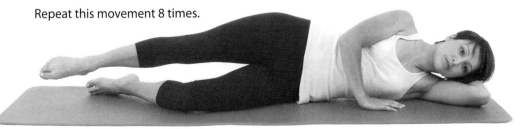

The Bridge Series

This series of exercises strengthens the gluteus maximus muscle, which is a powerful hip extensor muscle.

If you have an anterior pelvic tilt during rest, then strengthening this muscle is important to correct any muscle imbalances that you may have, which could be contributing to spinal instability and pain.

Teaching Points

You may find that your hamstrings feel as though they are going to cramp with this exercise. This indicates that you do not have effective firing of the glutes and that your hamstrings are trying to control the movement. As we often have tight hamstrings they may cramp as you perform this movement. It can help to stretch the hamstrings before this exercise.

If you have weak gluteal muscles, then you need to correct this imbalance by squeezing the buttocks muscles together as though you are holding a one dollar bill between the cheeks of your buttocks as you lift! This will encourage your buttocks to work throughout the movement.

You can prepare for the bridge series with the pelvic curl into back curl in the mobility section.

The leg lift bridge challenges the gluteus medius muscle, which is a pelvic stability challenge. This exercise prepares you for the full shoulder bridge.

To Prepare

Lie on your back with your knees bent. Tilt the pelvis back so that the small of your back presses into the floor. Keep your shoulders relaxed and away from the ears. Avoid tensing in the rib cage.

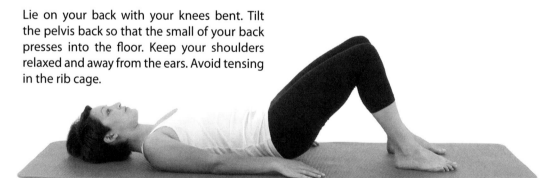

Bridge with Arm Overs

1. Exhale as you move from the tilt to a lift. The pelvis and back will lift up. Your back will be off the floor so that you are resting on your shoulder blades. Maintain the posterior tilt throughout the movement to protect the back.

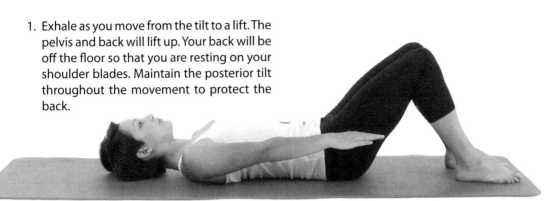

2. Inhale to take your arms up and over the body toward the head, ensuring that you do not lift from the rib cage.

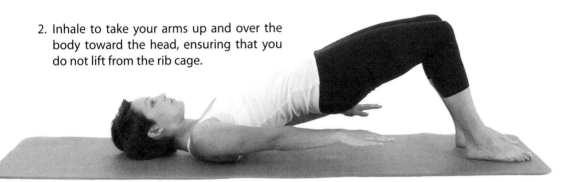

3. Exhale to bring the arms back, keeping the buttocks up and not letting them drop down!

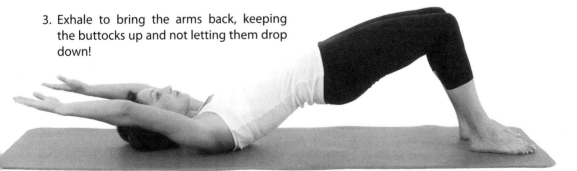

4. As the arms hover just above the floor, lower the pelvis back down to the floor. Repeat this movement 8 times.

Bridge Lowers

1. Exhale as you move from the tilt to a lift. The pelvis and back will lift up. Your back will be off the floor so that you are resting on your shoulder blades. Maintain the posterior tilt throughout the movement to protect the back.

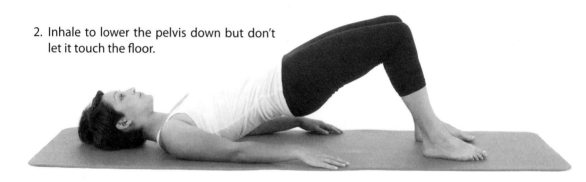

2. Inhale to lower the pelvis down but don't let it touch the floor.

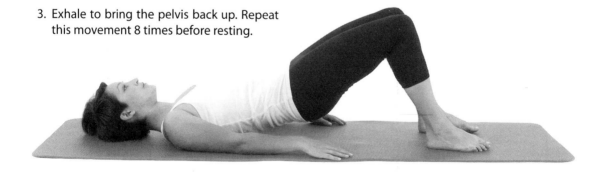

3. Exhale to bring the pelvis back up. Repeat this movement 8 times before resting.

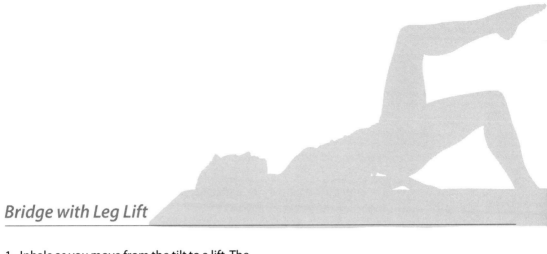

Bridge with Leg Lift

1. Inhale as you move from the tilt to a lift. The pelvis and back will lift up. Your back will be off the floor so that you are resting on your shoulder blades. Maintain the posterior tilt throughout the movement to protect the back.

2. Exhale to lift one leg into single leg lift. Inhale to lower. Keep the pelvis still throughout the movement.

You can make this movement harder by only lifting the feet 2 inches off the floor before lowering.

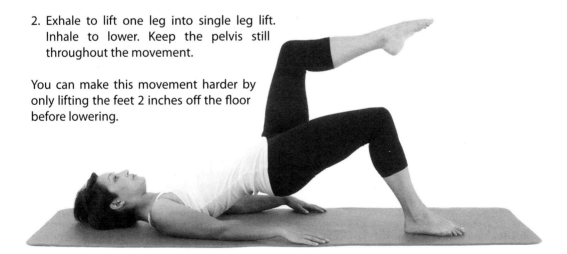

Swimming

The swimming movement involves hip and shoulder movements. It targets the buttocks muscle and helps to improve shoulder awareness, which will improve posture.

Teaching Points

Make sure that your lower back does not take the strain with this exercise by tucking your tailbone under to flatten the back during the movement.

If you feel that your shoulders lift toward the ears, as you bring your arm off the floor, keep your elbows bent to a 90-degree position.

You can keep your face resting on the floor to take the strain from the neck.

To make this exercise harder, do the movements faster while changing in the air and aim for 5 changes to each breath.

To Prepare:

Lie face down with your arms outstretched above your head. Keep your shoulders down away from the ears and your back away from the floor. Look down toward the floor with your chin tucked in and lift the head two inches off the floor. Tuck your tailbone under to prevent the back from arching. Tighten the deep abdominal muscles.

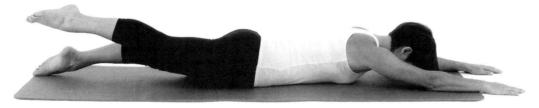

Single Leg Swimming

1. Exhale as you reach one leg away from the body and lift the leg from the hip. Be careful not to lift too high or the back may arch and take the strain. Inhale to lower.

2. Repeat the movement on the other leg and do 8 movements on each leg.

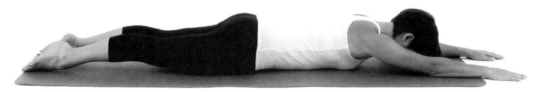

Single Arm Swimming

1. Keeping your shoulders away from the ears, exhale as you lift one arm up off the floor. Inhale to lower.

2. Repeat the movement on the opposite arm.

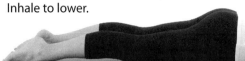
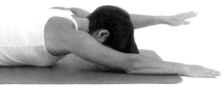

Arm & Leg Swimming

1. Inhale as you reach and lift one leg from the hip and the opposite arm up and away from the body. Keep your shoulders relaxed and move from the shoulder blades. Exhale to lower and change to lift the other side.

2. Try doing 2 or 3 changes to each breath and then continue for 8 sets.

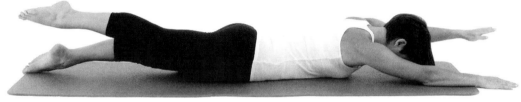

Double Leg Change

1. Inhale as you reach one leg away from the body and lift the leg from the hip. Exhale to bring the other leg up in the same way as you lower the first leg, changing legs in the air.

2. Repeat for 2 or 3 movements on the same exhalation, then inhale for 2 or 3 movements.

3. Continue for 8 sets of changes.

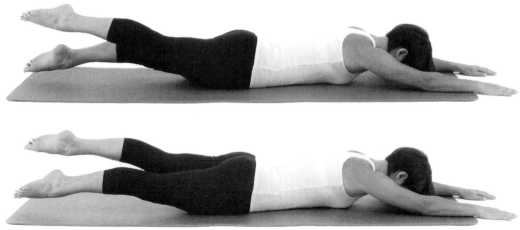

4-Point Reach

This exercise requires good pelvic control and scapular stability.

The 4-point reach improves balance and requires coordination.

Teaching Points

It is good to use a mirror with this movement to ensure that you do not lose the preparatory position throughout the exercise.

When you reach one arm forward, put your weight down through the opposite arm and the leg on the same side to balance your weight. Do the same with the legs. It should then be easier to proceed.

Begin the reach by keeping contact with the floor. If you still have control after the reach, then you can add the lift. Think about reaching away so that the focus is not simply on lifting but on reaching and lifting the leg up with control.

Be careful not to reach too far or your shoulders and/or hips will drop before you even attempt the lift.

To advance this movement you can hold the reach before you rest, keeping opposite limbs in the air but maintaining a level spine throughout. Hold for about 10 seconds and slowly build this to 30 seconds.

To Prepare

Come onto all fours so that your back is level, your hands are under your shoulders and your knees are under your hips. Keep your chin tucked in with the back of your head lifted toward the ceiling. Keep the shoulders away from the ears. Find your neutral spine and engage your deep abdominals.

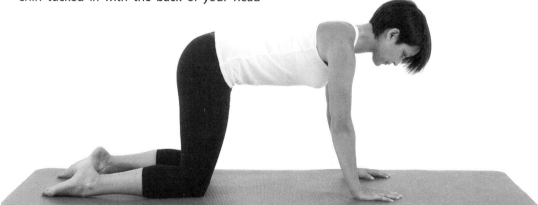

Single Arm Reach

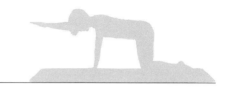

1. Keeping the shoulder blades still, keep contact with the floor, exhale and reach one arm forward. Don't lift the shoulder to the ear or tip the body to one side.

2. Inhale to hold and then exhale to gently float the arm up.

Repeat on the opposite side. Continue for 4 movements on each side.

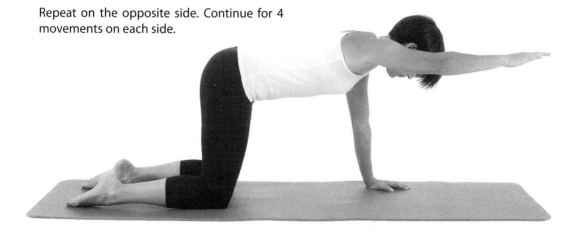

Single Leg Reach

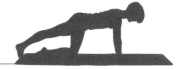

1. Keeping the pelvis level, exhale as you reach one leg away from the body, and keeping the leg low, inhale to hold.

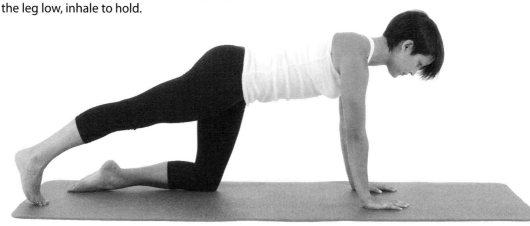

2. Exhale again as you lift the leg but do not allow the back to arch or the pelvis to tip. Inhale to lower the leg and return. Repeat on the other side. Continue for 4 movements on each side.

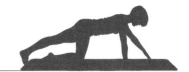

1. Maintaining the preparatory position, exhale to reach the left arm forward and, at the same time, reach the right leg backward.

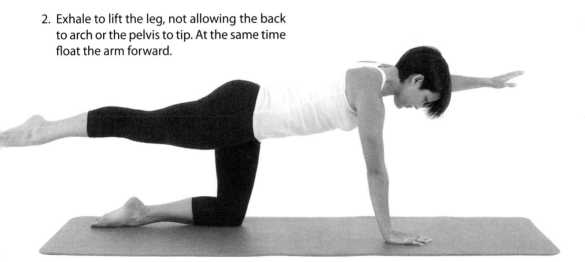

2. Exhale to lift the leg, not allowing the back to arch or the pelvis to tip. At the same time float the arm forward.

3. Inhale to lower the leg and return the arm back to the starting position. Repeat on the other side. Continue for 4 movements on each side.

Prone Leg Pull

This exercise challenges pelvic stability with movements of the hip to strengthen the muscles of the buttocks. Your core abdominals need to control the movement to keep the spine in neutral.

Teaching Points

This exercise requires you to keep your pelvis level throughout the movement to prevent you arching your back and tipping to one side. Imagine a glass of water resting in the small of the back. As you lift one leg you do not want to spill the glass of water!

Stretch the back of the leg before you lift the leg as this creates the "pull" effect.

The harder level, with both legs extended, requires abdominal strength to hold the position while you challenge yourself with movements of the hip to target the buttocks.

The full prone leg pull also requires good stability of the shoulder blades. Throughout the exercise, think about keeping the chin tucked in to strengthen the deep muscles of the neck.

This exercise will strengthen the stabilizing gluteus medius muscle on the supporting side and the powerful gluteus maximus muscle on the moving side to extend the hip.

It is important to extend the leg only from the hip. If you lift the leg too high you may arch your back and feel the pelvis tilt forward. Use a mirror to make sure you are moving correctly.

You can advance from the full leg pull to the twist and side bend.

To Prepare

Start in 4-point kneeling. Keep your knees under your hips and your hands under your shoulders. Do not let the head drop forward. Check that you are in neutral spine, your back should not be arched and you should relax between your shoulder blades.

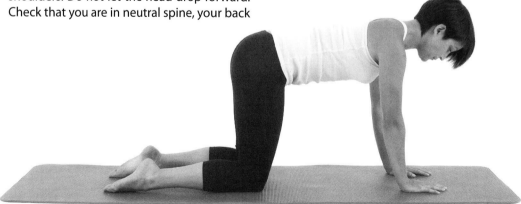

The Prone Leg Pull

1. Keeping the foot in contact with the floor, exhale to reach the leg away from the body, without losing the position of the back. Inhale to hold the stretch.

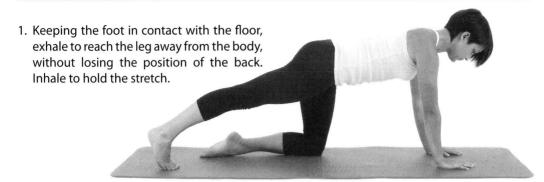

2. Exhale to gently lift the leg, being careful not to let the back arch.

   Return the leg and then repeat on the other side. Repeat for 8 lifts on each side.

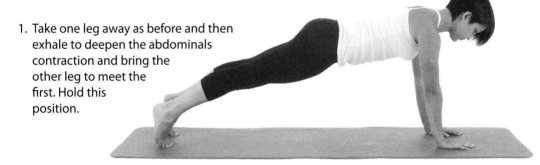

The Full Leg Pull

1. Take one leg away as before and then exhale to deepen the abdominals contraction and bring the other leg to meet the first. Hold this position.

2. Exhale now to lift one leg, as you did previously, without losing the neutral spine. Inhale to lower.

   Exhale to repeat on the other side. Repeat up to 8 times on each side.

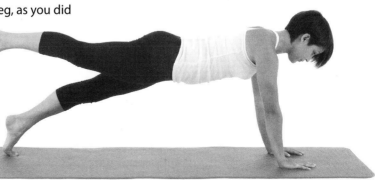

Criss Cross

This abdominal workout focuses on the obliques. The oblique muscles frame the rectus abdominus, the six-pack muscles. When the obliques are toned, they will pull in your waistline helping you to achieve an hourglass figure.

The obliques play a part in stabilizing the posture but they also assist flexion and rotation of the spine.

Teaching Points

You must maintain scapular stability throughout this exercise. Do not allow the shoulder blades to lift up toward the ears or to roll forward.

This exercise also works the muscles at the front of the hips. You must work to keep the pelvis stable throughout to prevent lifting. This challenges pelvic stability.

To Prepare

Lie on your back in a neutral spine position. Place your hands behind your head but don't link the fingers. Keep your elbows wide and the shoulders down, away from the ears and open across the front of the chest. Bend one knee into your chest and reach the other leg out along the mat.

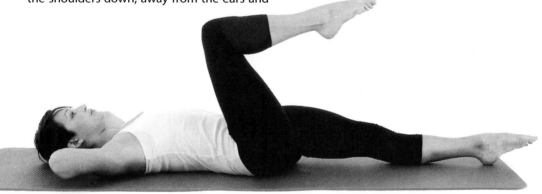

1. Exhale to curl to the side away from the straight leg, so that your shoulder is coming up toward the bent knee.

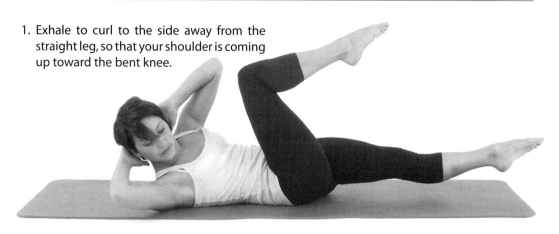

2. Inhale to stay high and exhale to change to the other side, swapping legs at the same time.

Hold and inhale, exhale to change again. Maintain the length of the torso throughout the movement.

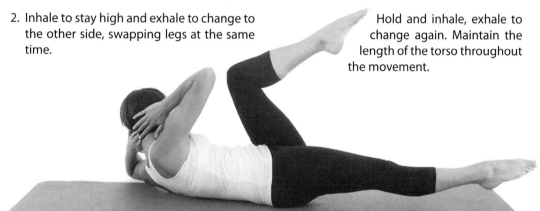

Working up to the Criss Cross

To Prepare

Lie on your back in a neutral spine position. Place your hands behind your head but don't link the fingers. Keep your elbows wide and the shoulders down, away from the ears and open across the front of the chest. Bend both knees so your feet are flat on the floor.

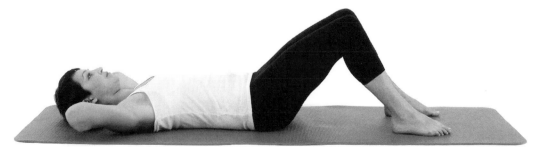

Oblique Curl

1. Exhale to curl up off the floor so that your shoulder is coming up toward the opposite knee. Inhale to lower.

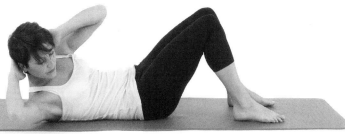

2. Repeat on the opposite side. Continue for 8 curls.

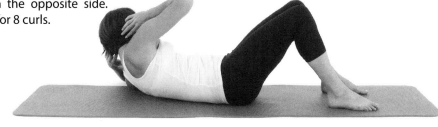

Sustained Oblique Curl

1. Exhale to curl up off the floor to a curl-up position. Inhale to hold.

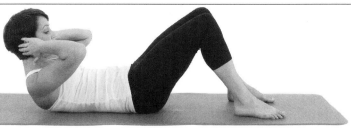

2. Exhale to move to one side. Inhale to hold.

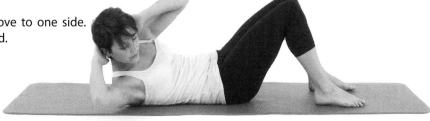

3. Sustaining the curl and keeping the pelvis level, exhale to move the upper body to the opposite side, maintaining the lift through the upper body.

4. Inhale to hold, exhale to change again. Continue for 8 movements to each side.

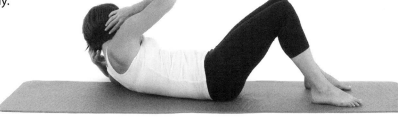

Sustained Oblique Curl from Double Tabletop

1. Come into a double tabletop position and exhale to come into the curl up. Inhale to hold.

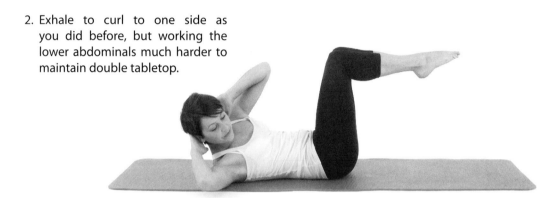

2. Exhale to curl to one side as you did before, but working the lower abdominals much harder to maintain double tabletop.

3. Inhale to hold and then exhale to move the upper body across to the other side, keeping the pelvis still throughout. Inhale to hold and then exhale to move in the opposite direction. Repeat 8 times.

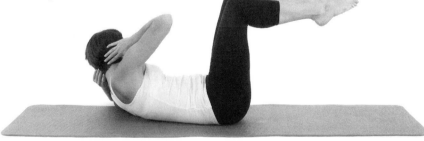

Floating Arms

This exercise is beneficial to address poor posture. It is an important exercise to raise awareness of your posture and how you can correct it.

Teaching Points

This exercise can be performed in a standing, lying or sitting position.

It is important with this series of exercises to use a mirror to check your shoulder positioning. Begin with small movements and only move one arm at a time initially.

At first you will probably only be able to take one arm just past your forehead. If you bring your arm too high or too far back, then you have probably compensated and lifted from the top of the shoulders.

Be careful not to lift your ribs. They should stay relaxed and not lift throughout the movement.

To Prepare

Stand with good posture.

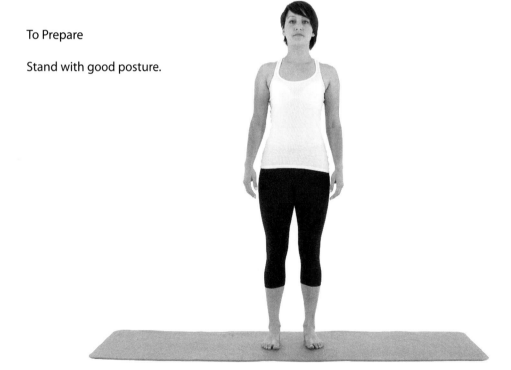

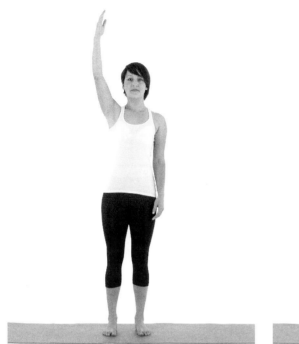

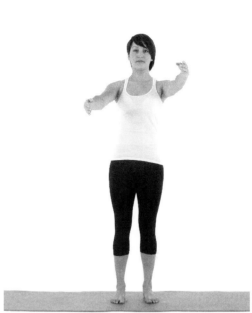

1. Exhale to float one arm up toward the ceiling, keeping your shoulders relaxed and not letting your rib cage lift.

2. Inhale to lower the arm down as you begin to move the other arm up. Exhale as the arms cross, and continue the movement.

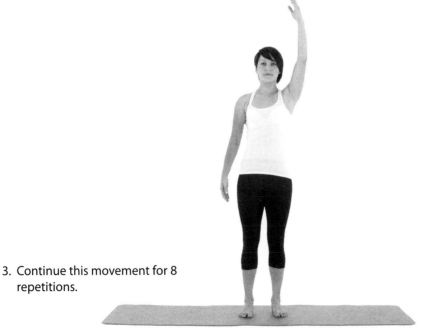

3. Continue this movement for 8 repetitions.

This series of movements encourages scapular control and improves upper body posture.

Teaching Points

It is important to begin the movements with small circles. You can increase the size of the circles as you improve your control.

The main area of correction with this exercise is to keep your rib cage soft. Also, be careful not to allow your shoulders to lift up toward your ears. Begin so that your shoulders are set in the correct position and maintain this posture throughout the move.

The same movements can be carried out lying on your side, back or standing up. On your back, you should feel your shoulder blades make contact with the floor as you move your arms. In side lying, it is easier to concentrate on not lifting the shoulders. In standing, keep a close eye on the rib cage. As the arms come up do not let the ribs hold tension and flare out.

This series prepares you for the double arm circle, which is an advanced exercise in the Contrology section.

Supine Arm Circles

To Prepare

Lying on your back in the resting position, draw the shoulders down away from the ears and lightly press the shoulders down into the floor, allowing the shoulder blades to rest on the floor. Now, keeping the shoulders set in this position, bring your arms up toward the ceiling.

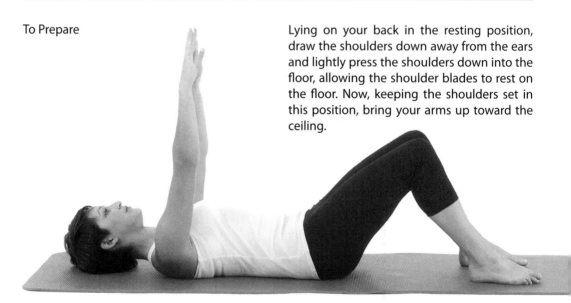

The Arm Circle

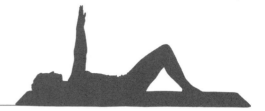

1. Exhale to take the arms back toward the head without losing the shoulder position and letting the rib cage lift.

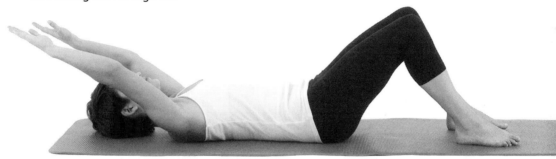

2. Inhale now to bring the arms around and back to the midline of the body. Repeat for 8 circles.

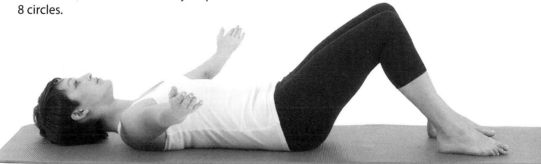

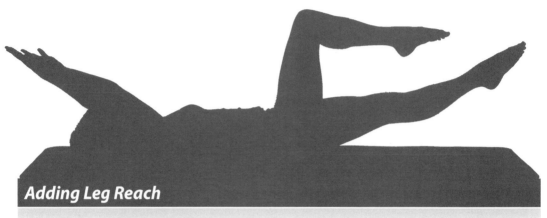

Adding Leg Reach

Only if you have control of the arm circle should you attempt to increase the challenge by adding lower limb movements.

Single Leg Reach

As you bring the arms behind you, reach one leg away. The leg reach challenges the neutral spine but will also cause the rib cage to lift earlier than with the arms alone. This move also challenges coordination.

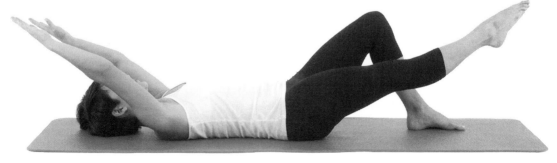

From Double Tabletop

If you can control double tabletop, then you can start from this position. As you exhale to bring the arms behind you, reach one leg away from double tabletop. This level really challenges the abdominals as well as scapular control.

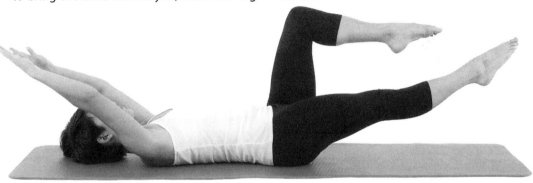

Double Leg Reach with Arm Circles

This advanced move requires full control of the core muscles as you reach both legs out while the arms circle. Be very careful not to tense in the upper body as you circle the arms and reach the legs out. Breathe out to reach away and inhale to return.

Side Lying Arm Circles

To Prepare

Lie on your side with a 3" head pillow. Your knees should be bent for support. Keep your top shoulder down, away from your ear and set the shoulder back so that it doesn't roll forward.

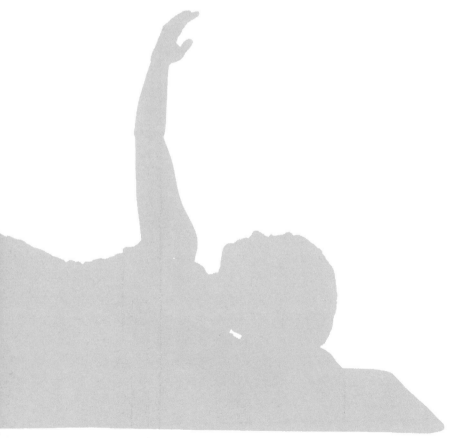

The Arm Circle

1. Inhale and begin the arm circle to bring the arm down toward the hips.

2. Exhale to control the shoulder position as you bring the arm behind you.

3. Now continue to move the arm up toward the head, again completing the circle. Repeat for 8 circles.

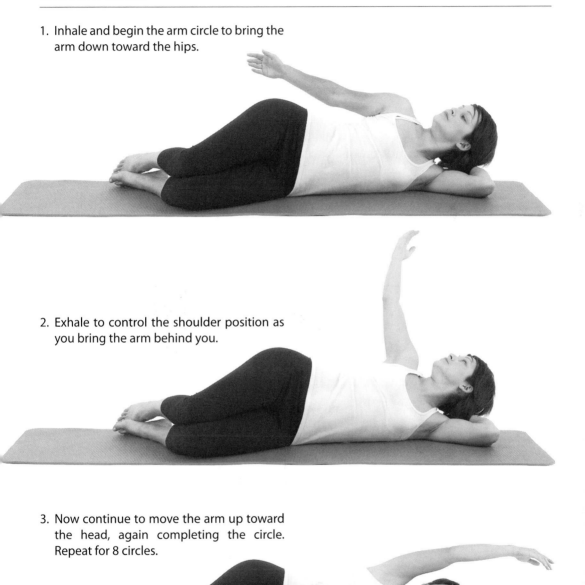

Arm Circles Standing

To Prepare

Standing in neutral spine, relax the shoulders
down toward the floor and let the shoulders
drop back, keeping the rib cage still.

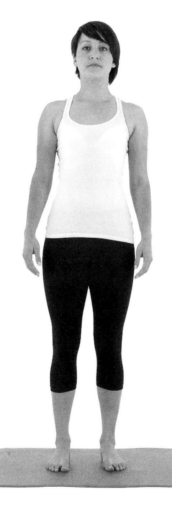

The Arm Circle

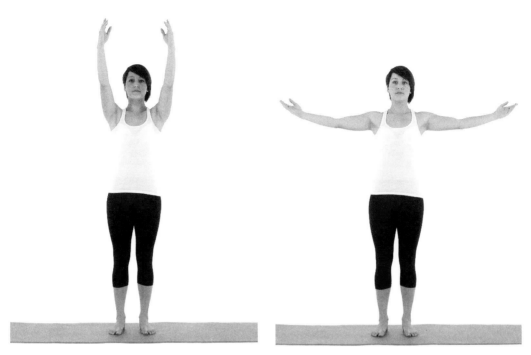

1. Exhale to lift both arms up to the midline of the body, without flaring in the rib cage or lifting the shoulders up.

2. Inhale to circle the arms around, keeping the arms in your peripheral vision.

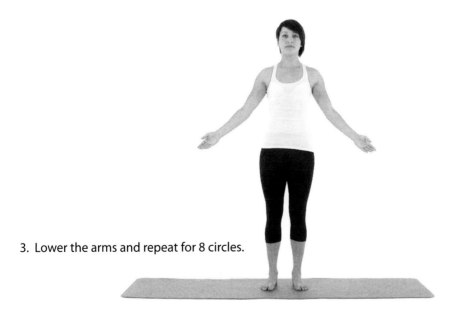

3. Lower the arms and repeat for 8 circles.

Upper Back Peel

This exercise encourages upper back extension and teaches good shoulder blade positioning.

It is an important exercise in any rehabilitation program for improving posture and reducing neck pain.

Teaching Points

You begin this movement by lifting the back of the head and keeping the chin tucked in. Imagine two pieces of string lifting the back of the head and the neck at the same time. Don't just lift the top of the head and look forward, or you will not strengthen the deep neck muscles responsible for supporting the head.

Be careful not to simply hinge from the lumbar spine with this exercise. The lower back should remain relaxed through this entire movement as you simply move from the back of the head and then the mid back. Keep your tailbone tucked under to prevent lumbar extension.

Keep your shoulder blades drawn down and back, squeezing the lower portion of the shoulder blades together throughout the movement.

You must understand this movement before you do the full back peel. The full back peel includes this upper back peel movement.

The upper back lift also advances this movement.

To Prepare

Lying on your front and looking down to the floor, have your arms at a 90-degree angle at your shoulders and elbows. Tuck your tailbone under to protect your lower back. Draw the shoulders down away from your ears and away from the floor.

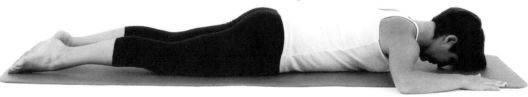

The Upper Back Peel

Exhale to lift from the back of the head up toward the ceiling, looking down throughout the movement. Keep the shoulders down and back. Continue the lift, so that you lift from the upper back, keeping your hands on the floor. Now inhale to lower back down.

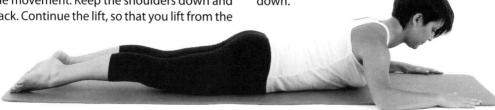

Upper Back Lift

This exercise requires you to lift the upper back off the floor to challenge thoracic extension. It is an exercise used in postural correction rehabilitation.

Teaching Points

This movement advances the upper back peel and is an alternative to the thoracic extension in sitting.

The upper back lift requires you to maintain the shoulder blade position as you lift from the upper back.

Make sure that you only lift from the mid and upper back, while your lower back remains relaxed. Keep your tailbone tucked under throughout the move.

To Prepare

Lying on your front and looking down to the floor, have your arms at a 90-degree angle at your shoulders and elbows. Tuck your tailbone under to protect your lower back. Draw the shoulders down, away from your ears and away from the floor.

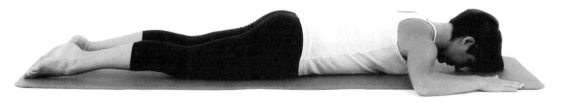

The Upper Back Lift

Exhale to lift the head and neck off the floor as you also lift the arms and upper back. Inhale to lower. Repeat for 8 lifts.

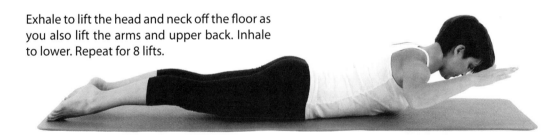

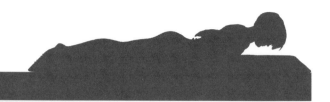

Prone Arm Lift

This movement strengths the lower trapezius muscle, which is important for correcting shoulder positioning and improving posture.

This exercise forms an important part of neck rehabilitation programs in postural correction.

Teaching Points

With the side arm lift and side glides, you must be careful not to lift up in the top of the shoulders as you will lose the benefit of the exercise. You must keep the shoulder position throughout.

You can keep your head resting on the floor throughout the exercise to make the movement easier on the neck. Start with simply bringing the shoulders down and back and then add the arm lift.

Keep the shoulders drawn toward one another throughout the movement. If you let the shoulders roll forward, then you will not feel the movement between the lower portion of the shoulder blades.

You could make this exercise harder by bringing the arms out further to the sides to a "T" position, but be careful not to lift the shoulders up toward the ears.

To Prepare

Lie on your front with your arms by your side, palms facing down. Tuck your tailbone under and bring your shoulders down and back, away from the ears and off the floor (setting the shoulder blades).

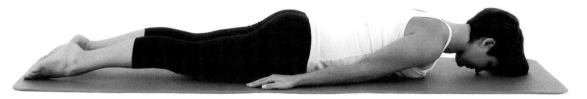

Side Arm Lift

1. Exhale to keep the shoulder position as you lift the arms and bring the face off the floor. Inhale to lower. Repeat 8 times.

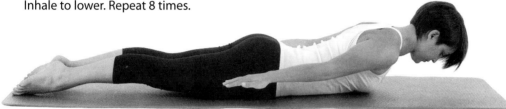

Side Arm Lift with added Side Glides

1. Exhale to lift the arms off the floor as before, keeping the shoulders peeled back. Inhale to hold.

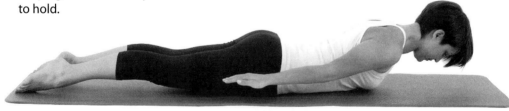

2. Exhale to bring the arms out to the sides to about 45 degrees not allowing the shoulders to lift. Inhale to bring the arms back to the sides again. Repeat for 8 movements.

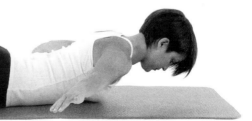

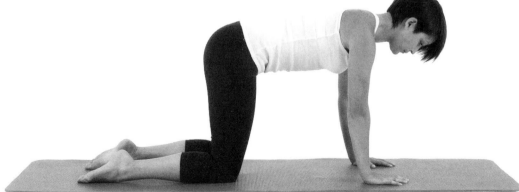

Push Up Prep

This movement strengthens the deep muscles that support the shoulder joint. It is also a good workout exercise for the arms.

Teaching Points

You must get the preparatory position right and then slowly move toward the floor as your elbows bend. Don't simply drop the head forward as you lower to the floor. Do not lose your neutral spine as you lower. It will be easier to simply push your buttocks up and arch your back as you lower, to save having any strain on your arms. However, will strain the back and will not target the right muscles. It is far more effective not to try and lower so far but keep the correct positioning.

The challenge comes when pushing back up. This is where you will need to exhale.

The push up prep prepares you for the full press up in the Controlology section (Chapter Seven).

To Prepare

Begin on all fours. Keep your knees under your hips to start and your arms under your shoulders. Keep your neck lengthened and your head lifted in line with your spine. Relax between your shoulder blades and find your neutral spine.

The Push Up Prep

Exhale to bend the elbows as you lower the face toward the floor. Stop if you feel you may arch in the lower back or lose the shoulder position. Inhale to hold this position and then exhale to push back up as the arms straighten again.

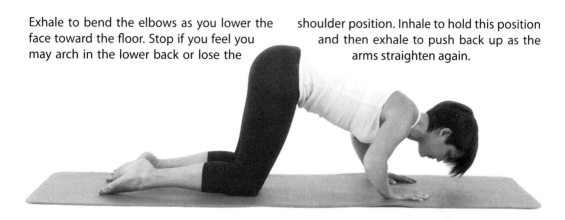

Progression

1. From the preparatory position, walk your hands forward, keeping your head over the top of your hands.

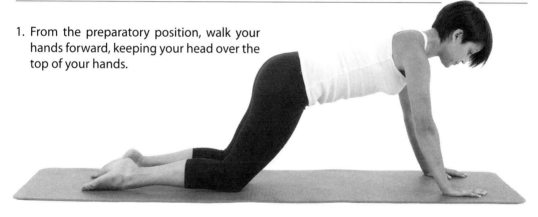

2. Inhale to lower from here and then exhale to push back up. Repeat 8 times.

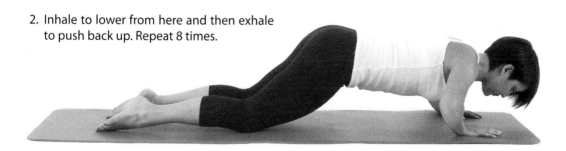

Thoracic Extensions

This exercise improves thoracic extension, which is often dominated by lumbar movement.

It is important to have a healthy thoracic spine to improve any problems that you may be suffering from in the cervical or lumbar spine.

Teaching Points

With thoracic extension, you will notice that you will not have very much movement, but remember that the thoracic spine is often stiff, especially into extension, as a result of our often flexed posture.

This exercise really is best performed in front of a mirror so that you can see that you are not cheating and overusing the lower back.

Thoracic extension can also be improved on your frontside with the upper back peel or lift.

Keep your chin tucked in to protect your neck with this move. You do not want your neck to overextend.

To Prepare

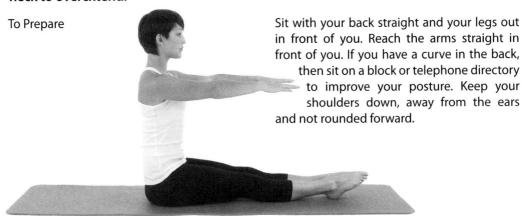

Sit with your back straight and your legs out in front of you. Reach the arms straight in front of you. If you have a curve in the back, then sit on a block or telephone directory to improve your posture. Keep your shoulders down, away from the ears and not rounded forward.

The Thoracic Extension

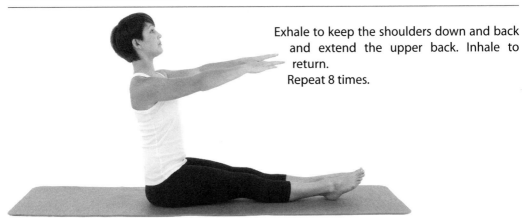

Exhale to keep the shoulders down and back and extend the upper back. Inhale to return.
Repeat 8 times.

Side Stretch

This stretch lengthens the muscles in the back that are often tight through lack of mobility in our lifestyles.

Teaching Points

The side stretch can be performed while sitting with both your legs in front of you, your legs crossed or from an alternative position including kneeling or standing.

Good movement with this exercise is to reach past your knees when the exercise is performed from a standing position.

The side bend is an advanced version of this exercise found in the Contrology section.

The Side Stretch

Sitting with good posture, keep your pelvic bones facing forward as you reach one arm up to the ceiling.

Exhale to reach the arm to one side but not lifting up from the sitting bone on the side you are stretching. Hold for between 10 and 20 seconds. Inhale to return and then repeat to the opposite side. Repeat for 4 stretches on each side.

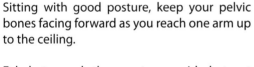

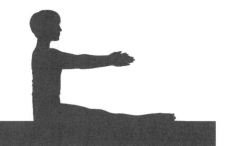

Bow and Arrow

This is an exercise to improve thoracic rotation. It also stretches the pectoral muscles.

Teaching Points

You must keep your pelvic bones facing forward throughout this movement.

The bow and arrow exercise can be performed in standing or sitting. It is especially good for those with sedentary occupations.

The spine twist is another thoracic rotation exercise that can be advanced to the saw. The threading the needle movement also improves thoracic rotation.

Keep your shoulders down throughout this movement and keep your shoulders above your hips. Do not lean back.

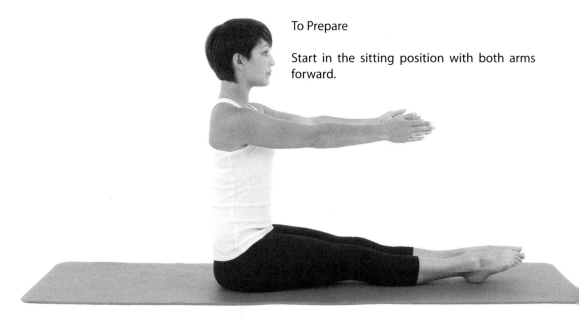

To Prepare

Start in the sitting position with both arms forward.

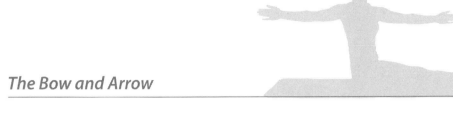

The Bow and Arrow

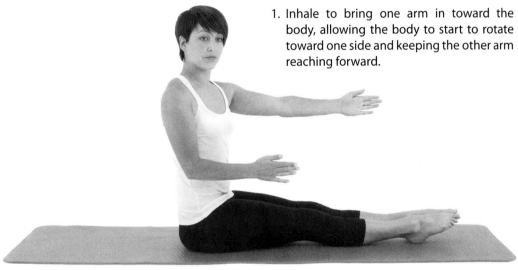

1. Inhale to bring one arm in toward the body, allowing the body to start to rotate toward one side and keeping the other arm reaching forward.

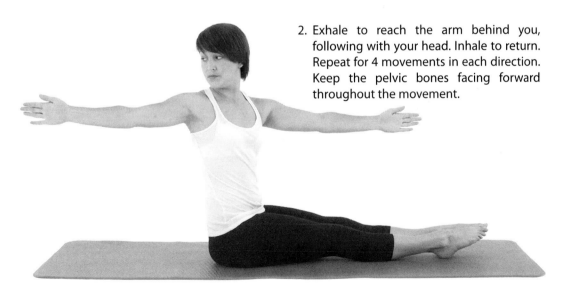

2. Exhale to reach the arm behind you, following with your head. Inhale to return. Repeat for 4 movements in each direction. Keep the pelvic bones facing forward throughout the movement.

Controlled Over Shrug

This exercise controls scapular (shoulder blade) position as you move the arms over your head.

Teaching Points

It is important not to try to achieve the full movement if you are losing control and lifting in the top of the shoulders as you bring your arms up. Typically, we tend to lift in the upper trapezius muscle too early in the movement and so you need to do this exercise in front of a mirror in order to check your posture throughout.

To Prepare

Sit with good posture, arms open to the side.

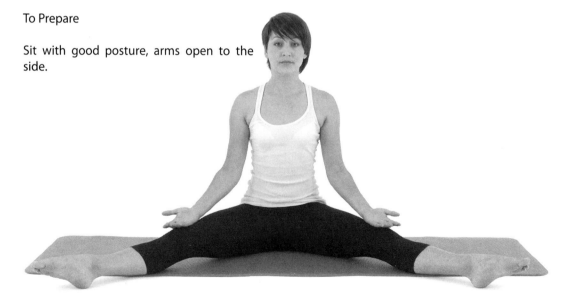

The Over Shrug

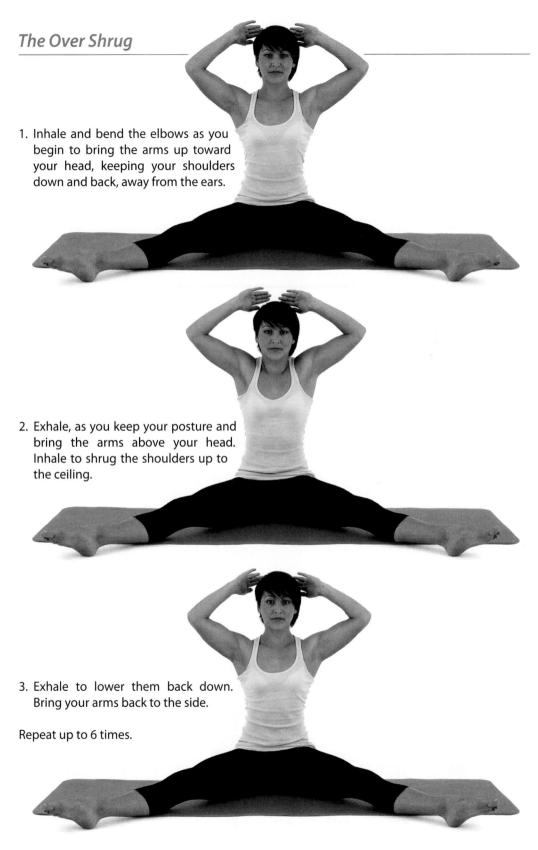

1. Inhale and bend the elbows as you begin to bring the arms up toward your head, keeping your shoulders down and back, away from the ears.

2. Exhale, as you keep your posture and bring the arms above your head. Inhale to shrug the shoulders up to the ceiling.

3. Exhale to lower them back down. Bring your arms back to the side.

Repeat up to 6 times.

Pelvic Tilt into Back Curl

This exercise moves the spine from the lowest part of the back, the tailbone, to the mid back adjacent to your shoulder blades.

The pelvic tilt and back curl are important movements for improving mobility in the back but these movements also strengthen the buttocks muscle, the gluteus maximus. It is a common rehabilitation exercise for low back pain and often eases back pain caused by immobility.

Teaching Points

Place your hands to form a diamond below the belly button so that your thumbs are pointing toward your belly button and your fingers toward your pubic bone. If you imagine a marble in the center of the diamond, you want to roll the marble toward your thumbs as you rotate your pelvis backward, lifting the pubic bone up. Now as you continue to peel from the floor, the marble must stay rolled toward your thumbs. Do not level the pelvis again until the movement is completed.

Imagining that your spine represents a string of pearls, peel the spine from the floor so that the bones of the back come away from the mat, one at a time, much like the pearls on the necklace will move as you lift the string from one end.

The strength component of this exercise can be challenged with the bridge series. The mobility component can be challenged with the roll back.

To Prepare

Start in the resting position.

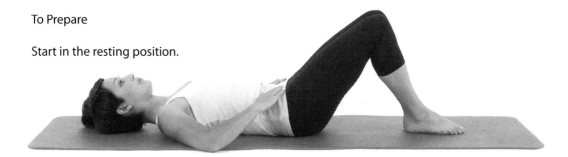

The Pelvic Tilt

Inhale to flatten the small of your back into the floor by tilting the pelvis backward so that your tailbone comes off the floor.

The Back Curl

Exhale to continue to peel the back from the floor up to your shoulders. Inhale at the top of this movement and then exhale to peel back down. Repeat for 8 curls.

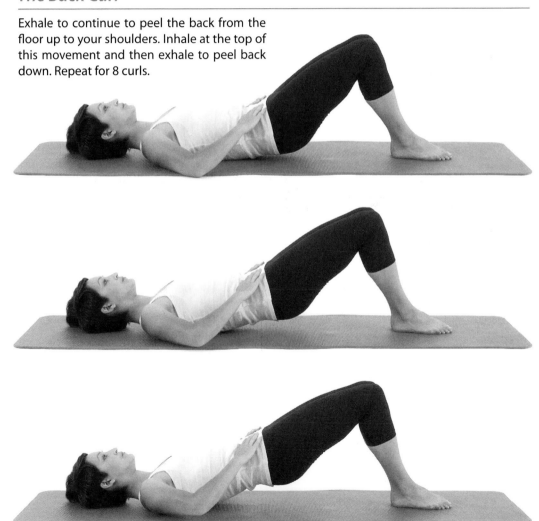

Full Back Peel

The full back peel continues from the upper back peel to mobilize the entire back, from the neck through to the lumbar spine. It is an important exercise to promote extension of the spine and a healthy back.

Teaching Points

It is important to include the upper back peel in this movement so that you do not simply hinge from the most mobile part of your back.

If you are stiff in your lower back, you may feel that you cannot extend in the lower back and that, after the shoulders lift, the pelvic bones will raise while not actually mobilizing the spine at all. If this is the case, you cannot come up as high. Always keep the pelvic bones in contact with the floor. Think about where the muscle activity is coming from in the back. As soon as you feel tension in the lower back you have come up as high as you should be coming up.

When peeling up from the front, you need to visualize lifting first your face from the floor, then your chest followed by your ribcage and finally your navel. Viewed from behind, your head will leave the floor first, then your shoulders and upper back, followed by your mid back and shoulder blades and finally the lower back.

To Prepare

Lie on your front with your arms out to the sides and your elbows bent to 90 degrees. Now tuck your tailbone under to protect your lower back. Look down with your chin tucked in.

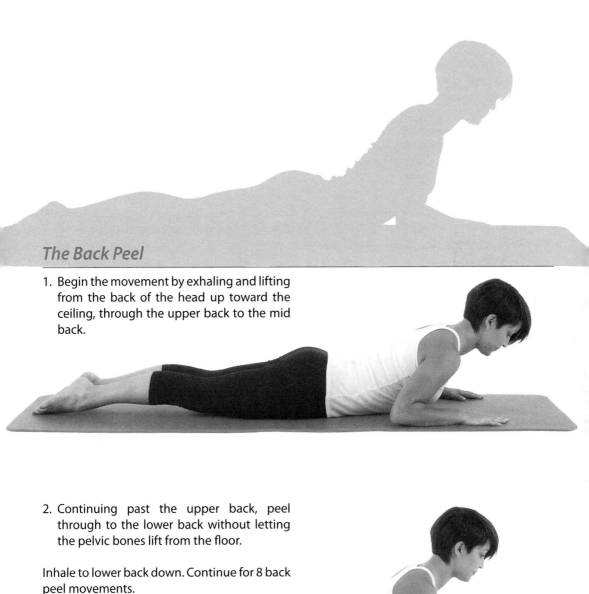

The Back Peel

1. Begin the movement by exhaling and lifting from the back of the head up toward the ceiling, through the upper back to the mid back.

2. Continuing past the upper back, peel through to the lower back without letting the pelvic bones lift from the floor.

Inhale to lower back down. Continue for 8 back peel movements.

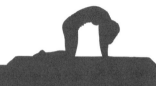

The Cat Stretch

This is an exercise that is typically seen in the world of yoga. It stretches the spine and relaxes the muscles in the back that are often tight.

Teaching Points

Keep this exercise within the range that you are comfortable with. This exercise should relax the back, so do not overstretch.

Use your abdominal muscles to control the movement.

Keep your neck moving with the rest of the back. The movement should flow like a rippled effect, from the tailbone to the head.

To Prepare

Start in 4-point kneeling. Your knees should be under your hips and your hands under your shoulders. Relax between your shoulder blades. Engage your deep abdominal muscles and keep the back of your head lifted toward the ceiling.

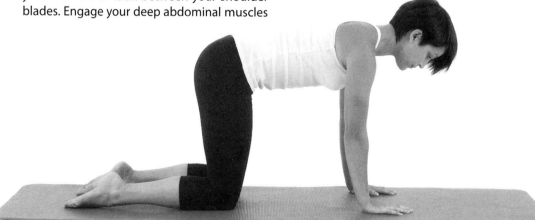

The Cat Stretch

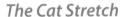

1. Inhale to tuck your tailbone under and bring your chin to your chest, lifting the back up toward the ceiling.

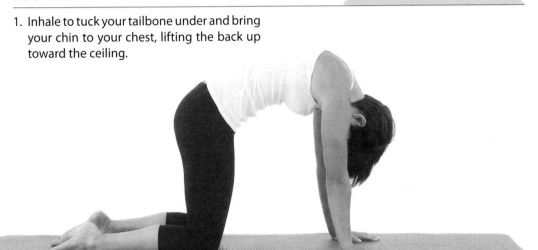

2. Exhale to tilt the pelvis forward as you push the tailbone gently up toward the ceiling while looking up and relaxing between the shoulder blades.

Now move into the opposite direction and repeat for 8 movements.

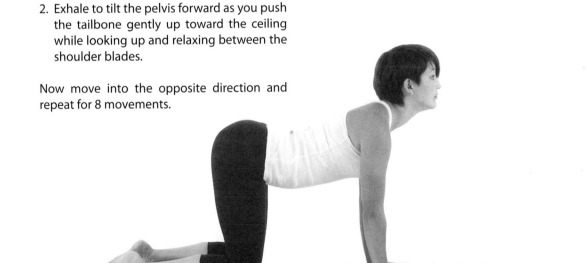

Thread the Needle

This is a thoracic rotation exercise. It mobilizes the stiffest part of the back.

Teaching Points

Thoracic rotation is particularly important if you spend a lot of the day sitting, including driving. Our thoracic spines tend to tighten and we need to practice rotation to keep the spine healthy and moving.

You must keep the pelvis level as you rotate the upper back. Imagine a glass of water resting on the low back. Be careful not spill this water during the movement.

Bend the arm on the side you are rotating toward, as though you are performing a one armed push up. This will allow you to get more rotation.

Rotation is also targeted with the spine twist and the saw movements.

To Prepare

Start in 4-point kneeling in neutral spine, with the back of your head lifted up toward the ceiling and your shoulders relaxed. Engage your deep abdominals.

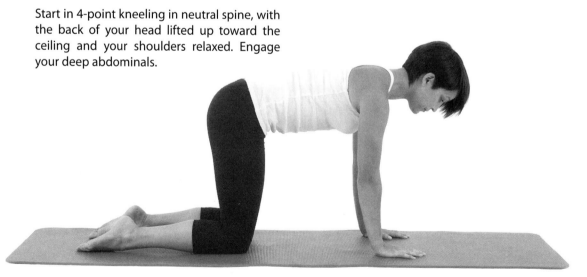

Threading the Needle

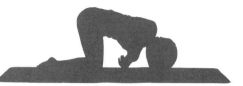

1. Lift one arm off of the floor and exhale as you take your lifted arm under the opposite arm, rotating the upper body only.

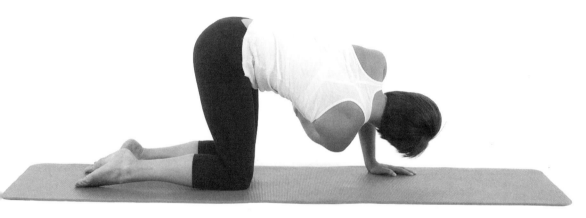

2. Inhale to return to the start position and repeat on the other side.

Do 8 rotations in total, 4 to each side.

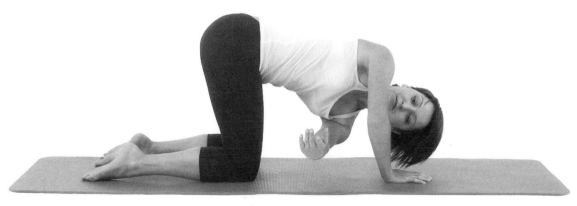

Spine Twist

This is a thoracic rotation exercise that, if performed with the legs straight, also lengthens the hamstrings.

Teaching Points

Imagine that your pelvic bones are spotlights and that these spotlights must stay pointing forward throughout the movement.

It is important to move only from the mid back so you must isolate your movement to this part of the back. Have your arms stretched to the sides and imagine you have a broomstick behind you and that your arms are tied to this broomstick as you rotate. If you do not use this visualization, then one arm tends to come forward of the body, and if this occurs you will not be localizing movement to the thoracic spine.

If your arms feel too heavy when they are stretched to the side, you can bend your elbows and bring your arms in front of the body.

Keep lifted through the top of the head for this exercise, as though a helium balloon is lifting the back of the head.

This movement can also be performed while standing but it is then easier to move from the hips so you will need to focus on keeping the pelvis still throughout the movement.

Keep your shoulders relaxed throughout the movement. Do not hold tension in the upper body.

The saw movement in the Contrology section advances the spine twist by adding a reach after the twist.

To Prepare

Sit with your legs extended out in front but just wider than the body. Sit tall so that your spine is in neutral and you have good upper body posture.

You may need to sit on a block to ensure you can achieve and maintain neutral. Straighten the arms out to the sides.

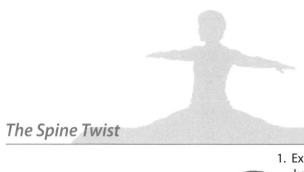

The Spine Twist

1. Exhale to rotate the body to one side, keeping the pelvic bones facing forward. Stop when you feel that you need to move from the hips to get further.

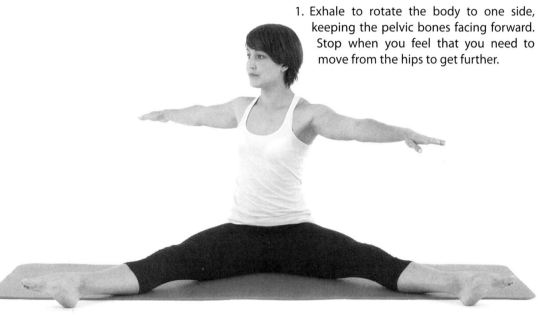

2. Inhale to return to the front and then exhale to repeat to the other side.

Repeat 4 times in each direction.

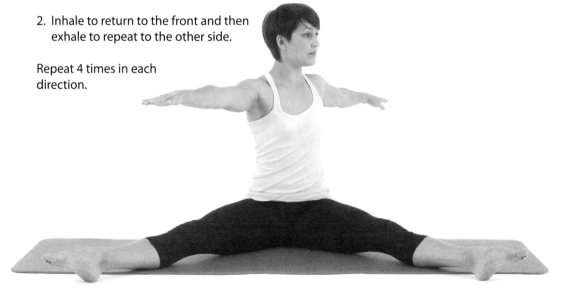

Open Leg Balance

The open leg balance is a very difficult exercise that challenges balance. It requires good hamstring length and strong abdominal and thigh muscles.

Teaching Points

With this exercise you must keep a neutral spine. Try to keep the back as straight as you can without losing the upper body posture by lifting in the shoulders or flexing forward.

If you find the exercise too difficult, try to work out what is limiting you. If it is abdominal strength, then work through the spinal stability section to address your weakness or, if you are tight in the hamstrings, practice the hamstring stretch or the spine stretch forward, to improve length.

Once you have corrected the open leg balance and the rocker prep, you can advance to the open leg rocker.

To Prepare

Sit with your knees bent and your hands holding onto your ankles. Keep your spine in neutral, which will be slightly lifted through the back. Relax your shoulders and engage your abdominal muscles.

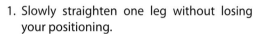

The Open Leg Balance

1. Slowly straighten one leg without losing your positioning.

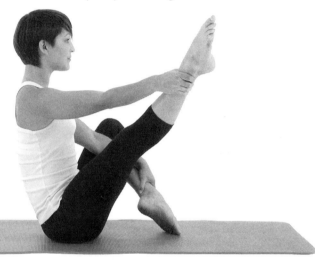

2. Exhale now to straighten the other leg as well, keeping the back straight and your shoulders relaxed. Hold this position for between 10 to 30 seconds.

3. Now bring one leg down at a time to relax.

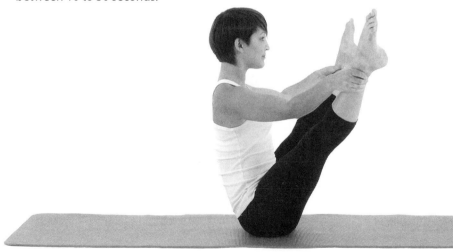

The rocker prep requires movement of the lower spine to initiate the roll back and control of the core muscles not to move too far and to return to the start position. You must keep the shoulders relaxed throughout.

Teaching Points

It is important to relax the shoulders throughout this movement as you will probably find that the shoulders want to lift up.

The rocker prep is a small movement with just enough backward tilt of the pelvis to initiate a roll back, then a bend (flex) in the lumbar spine to deepen the curve of the spine. A contraction of the abdominals and extension of the spine brings you straighter and returns you to the starting position.

If this level is too difficult, then practice with your feet on the floor initially, to understand what the movement requires, before you advance by lifting the feet.

You can advance from the rocker prep to the rolling series; begin with the rolling like a ball in the Contrology section.

To Prepare

Sit with your knees bent and place your hands under your thighs. Relax your shoulders. Engage your deep abdominal muscles and lift your feet off the floor. Hold this position.

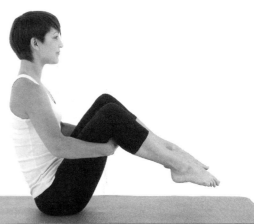

The Rocker Prep

Inhale to begin to tilt the pelvis in a backward direction and then exhale to continue the movement to deepen the curve of the lower back further and press the lowest part of the spine into the floor. Inhale to return to the starting position.

Repeat for 8 movements.

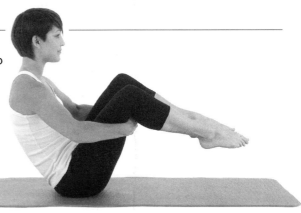

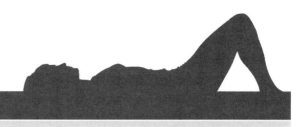

Knee Hug

This exercise stretches the muscles of the back and is great for stretching a stiff overworked spine.

Teaching Points

This stretch can be performed between exercises, before getting up in the mornings or just throughout the day to stretch the back.

You can stretch one knee at a time in toward your chest, if you feel that bringing in both knees is too much.

To Prepare

Lie on your back with your knees bent in the resting position.

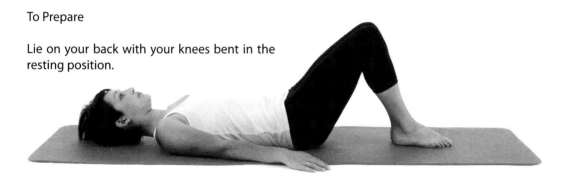

The Knee Hug

Gently bring one knee into the chest, supporting with your arms and then bring the other knee into meet the first. Hold the stretch as you relax the upper body and breathe. Hold for up to 30 seconds and then lower one leg at a time.

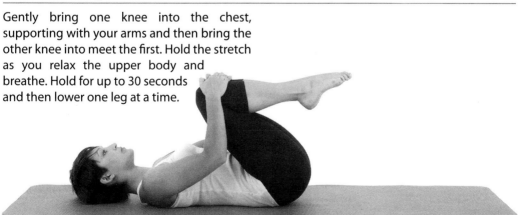

Roll Down

The roll down mobilizes the whole spine and stretches the hamstrings from a standing position. It is a movement that improves flexion of the spine.

The roll down is often used in a Pilates class as a warm up or warm down exercise and it should always feel comfortable.

Teaching Points

As you roll down you can relax the knees to lessen the pull on the hamstrings.

You can perform this movement from leaning against a wall to give extra feedback as to whether you are moving from all areas of the spine.

Be sure that you begin the movement by tucking your chin in toward the chest and then let your shoulders roll forward and down, not shrugging the shoulders up. As you finish the movement, you must roll the shoulders back into good posture and let the head lengthen again toward the ceiling.

The pelvis should tilt forward at the last part of the forward movement. Returning to a neutral spine, by tilting the pelvis backward, begins the return to a standing position.

If you have back pain that is made worse by moving forward, you should avoid this movement or simply work from the upper body only. Avoid moving from the lower back or tipping the pelvis forward.

To Prepare

Stand in neutral spine with good posture. Relax your arms by your sides.

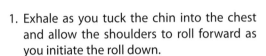

1. Exhale as you tuck the chin into the chest and allow the shoulders to roll forward as you initiate the roll down.

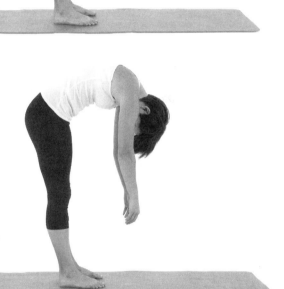

2. Continue the roll down by rolling through the upper back to the lower back.

3. Now allow the pelvis to tip forward.

4. Inhale to hold this position and then bend the knees slightly to stack the spine back to the starting position. Begin the return by tipping the pelvis backward to neutral and then, from the lower back to the upper back, stack the bones of the spine one on top of another, relaxing the shoulders and finishing in good posture.

Repeat up to 8 times

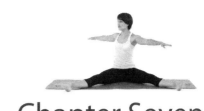

Chapter Seven
Original Contrology:

The Advanced Exercises

The Hundred

The Pilates Hundred is probably the most known of the Pilates matwork exercises.

This classic exercise builds strength, stamina and coordination. It requires you to combine the breath with movement. The hundred is often used as a warm-up exercise to get the blood pumping throughout your body.

The Hundred exercise integrates a number of movements, combined with core stability, giving your mind a number of issues to concentrate on. This teaches you to consciously optimize your body positioning and movement.

Teaching Points

The Hundred emphasizes lateral breathing. This is breathing into the sides of your lower rib cage. Try not to breathe from the upper chest.

You advance to the Hundred with the tabletop series. The exercise is made easier by working from the floor initially with just your arms moving, then from single tabletop to double, working through the tabletop series. Use the lower levels to perfect the breath before you make the challenge too advanced by reaching the legs away.

Do not attempt the full movement if you cannot control double table top reach in the tabletop series.

To Prepare

Lie on your back in the resting position. Exhale to come into the curl-up position. Inhale to hold and then exhale to straighten one leg at a time to a 45-degree angle, away from the body.

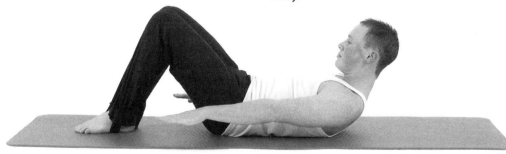

The Hundred Action

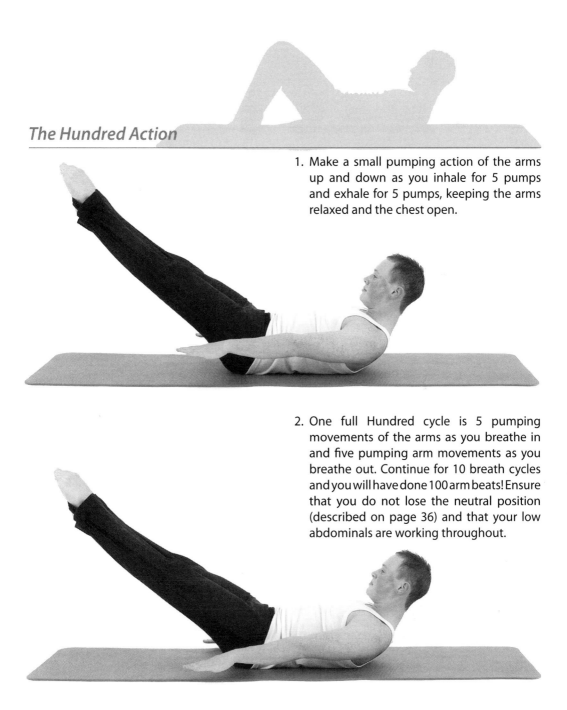

1. Make a small pumping action of the arms up and down as you inhale for 5 pumps and exhale for 5 pumps, keeping the arms relaxed and the chest open.

2. One full Hundred cycle is 5 pumping movements of the arms as you breathe in and five pumping arm movements as you breathe out. Continue for 10 breath cycles and you will have done 100 arm beats! Ensure that you do not lose the neutral position (described on page 36) and that your low abdominals are working throughout.

Scissors

The scissors exercise works the abdominal muscles hard as they are being challenged by the resistance of both legs moving in a scissor action.

The scissors movement also improves the length of the hamstrings and mobility of the hips.

Teaching Points

If your hamstrings are tight, you will need to lengthen the muscles with active stretches, such as the spine stretch or with the passive hamstring stretch and gently ease into the full scissor action.

You will work harder with this exercise if you perform the movement slowly.

Make sure that you are not swaying from one side to the other as you move the legs, keep the body centrally aligned and look directly between your legs throughout the movement.

You can advance to the full scissor from the scissor preps (bent knee scissors) in the rehabilitation exercises. With the legs straight the lever length is increased weight of the lower leg is heavier and therefore the load on the abdominals is greater.

To Prepare

Lie on your back in the resting position. Bring one leg toward you keeping the leg straight. Now straighten the other leg away from you, resting on the floor. Exhale to float this leg off the floor and come into a curl-up position.

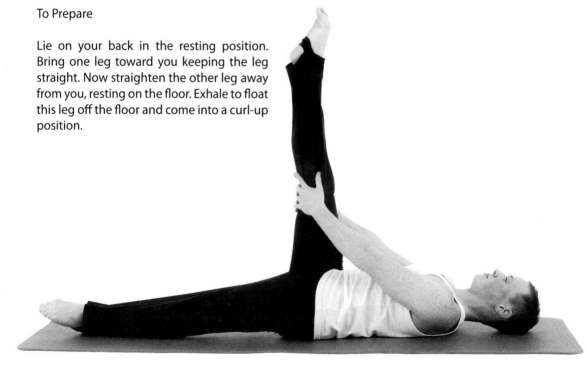

The Scissor Action

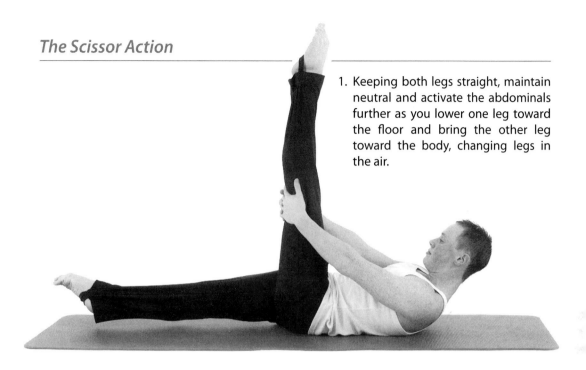

1. Keeping both legs straight, maintain neutral and activate the abdominals further as you lower one leg toward the floor and bring the other leg toward the body, changing legs in the air.

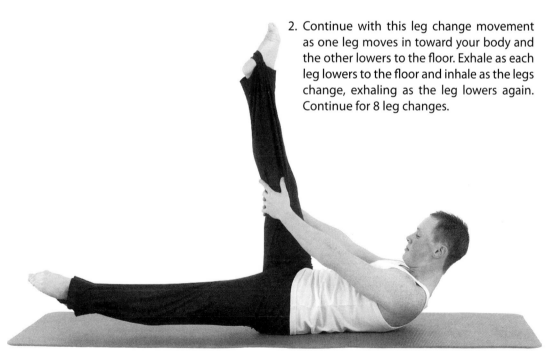

2. Continue with this leg change movement as one leg moves in toward your body and the other lowers to the floor. Exhale as each leg lowers to the floor and inhale as the legs change, exhaling as the leg lowers again. Continue for 8 leg changes.

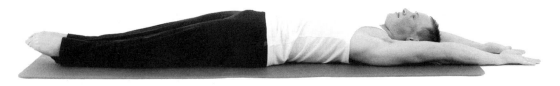

Roll Up

The roll up is one of Joseph Pilates' original mat exercises. The aim is to increase abdominal strength and articulation of the spine. It has been said that one Pilates roll up is equal to six regular sit ups and is much better than crunches for creating a flat stomach!

The roll up is also good for improving hamstring length.

Teaching Points

The most difficult part of the movement is the initiation of the roll up—coming up from the floor. If you feel that you are trying to swing yourself up, then first you need to improve your control and strength with the roll back and curl up exercises.

Do not try to lift too early with this exercise. As your arms come up over your head past your eyes you start to initiate the roll up movement. Your chin should be tucked in throughout the movement. You can keep your arms behind your head to reduce tension in your neck, but if you do this make sure that you do not push the head up.

It is important with this exercise not to overuse the hip flexors (the muscles at the front of the hips) as this will cause compression in the lower back. If you feel these muscles are overworking and that you are unable to keep your legs straight on the floor, return to the curl up or roll back exercise again.

The breath really helps you to control this exercise. Exhale slowly as you curl up and you will have more control and inner strength.

To Prepare

Lie on the floor with your legs straight and your arms by your sides. Relax your shoulders away from your ears. Leaving your shoulder blades anchored to the floor and keeping your ribs relaxed, bring your arms straight up over your head so that your fingertips are pointing to the wall behind you.

The Roll Up

1. Inhale as you bring your arms up over your head. As your arms pass your ears, let the chin drop and the head and upper spine join the motion to curve up.

2. Exhale now to continue in one smooth movement to roll your body in an "up and over" motion toward your toes. Keeping the head tucked, the abdominals activated and the back rounded, reach for your toes.

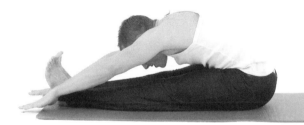

The Roll Back

Inhale to initiate the roll back, tuck the tailbone under and begin to curl back to the floor vertebrae by vertebrae. Keep the legs on the floor and don't let them lift up as you roll down. Check that your shoulders are relaxed and not lifting.

Exhale halfway back and continue to set one vertebrae after another down on the floor.

The key is to keep your upper body curve as you go down slowly and sequentially. Once your shoulders come to the floor, the arms go with the head as they reach back to starting position, the upper neck and head moving toward the floor.

Do up to 8 repetitions: The roll up and roll back is one continuous controlled flowing motion.

Single Leg Stretch

This abdominal strength exercise challenges the transversus abdominus muscle by working the rectus abdominus muscle and the lower limbs at the same time.

This movement teaches us to consciously perfect our body alignment while moving. This conscious awareness is important to achieve functional carry over of the benefits of working core stability with lower limb activity such as walking or running.

This exercise lengthens the abdominal muscles promoting a long, lean trunk. It also builds endurance of abdominal muscles. Improving endurance is really important in preventing and rehabilitating back pain. We also get an active stretch of the often tight hamstrings.

Teaching Points

Keep your shoulders relaxed through the movement and avoid rocking from side to side. Keep looking directly forward between your legs.

As you reach your leg away, be sure that you don't let your back arch. The further you reach your leg away, the heavier the leg will be and the harder it will be to control. Always work to maintain a neutral spine.

To prepare for this exercise, work through the leg reach series of the rehabilitation exercises and practice holding the curl-up movement.

To Prepare

Lying on your back, straighten one leg away from the body and bring one knee into the chest.

On the next exhalation, curl up and bring the extended leg 2 inches off the floor.

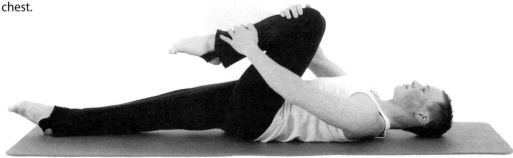

The Single Leg Stretch

1. Inhale and as you exhale reach the bent leg away, at the same time bringing the opposite leg into the chest.

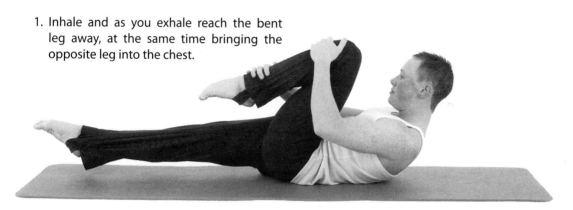

2. Continue changing legs, reaching the leg and lengthening through the body as you move. Keep your eyes focused between your legs. Keep your legs moving in a straight line.

Repeat for 8 movements on each leg.

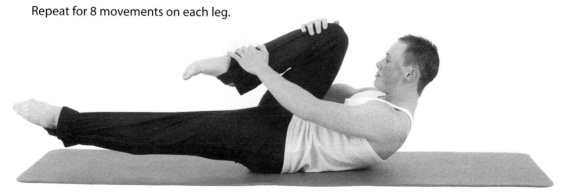

Double Leg Stretch

This is another good exercise for building abdominal endurance.

This exercise challenges concentration and core control by adding upper limb movements to lower limb movement from a curl-up position. It is an exercise that, when performed well, achieves mind-body control.

The arm movement of the double leg stretch begins to challenge scapular stability as you control upper body posture with arm movements.

Teaching Points

Moving both arms and legs away together challenges the deep abdominal muscle more than the single leg stretch, as you have doubled the weight by both of the legs being taken away. If this is too difficult, keep the legs closer to the body by not reaching away as far.

The lower you reach your legs the harder this movement is. If you reach higher, you will find the movement easier on the abdominals, but you will stretch the hamstrings more.

Keep your shoulders relaxed into the floor throughout the movement, and relax your rib cage. As you take your arms behind you, be sure that you do not allow the ribs to lift or the shoulders to tense.

Keep the arms in your peripheral vision. If you circle too wide, your shoulders will lift closer to the ears and you will overwork the already tight neck muscles.

Be careful not to strain the neck with this movement. Keep lifting up from the chest.

Advance to this exercise with the arm circles in supine in the scapular stability rehabilitation exercises.

To Prepare

Lying on your back, hug your knees into your chest. Inhale and curl the upper body up.

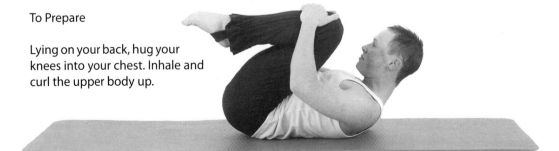

The Double Leg Stretch

1. Exhale and reach your legs and arms away from the body to a 45-degree angle.

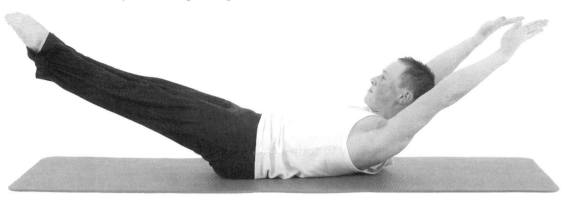

2. Inhale as you circle the arms around and bring your knees back into your chest.

Continue for up to 8 repetitions.

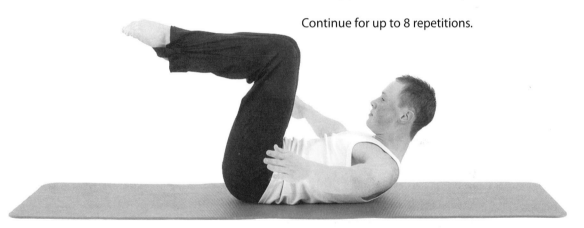

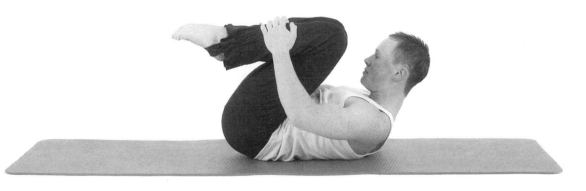

The Roll-Over

This is a difficult exercise that requires strength, control and mobility of the spine.

The spine is stretched as you lift one vertebrae at a time off the floor using the control and strength of the abdominal muscles.

Teaching Points

Performing this exercise with your knees bent makes it much easier.

Be very careful not to put too much weight on the neck as this can reduce the blood flow from the feet to the head and could injure the disks in the neck.

For this exercise you need advanced flexibility. If you are tight in your hamstrings, you will not be able to bring the legs as low to the floor as they move over your head. If your abdominals do not have the strength, you will not be able to control the movement and if you are stiff in the spine, you will not be able to initiate the movement.

To Prepare

Lie on your back with your arms by your side and your legs extended.

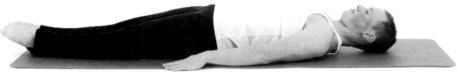

Inhale as you bring the legs to the ceiling, keeping the legs straight. Exhale.

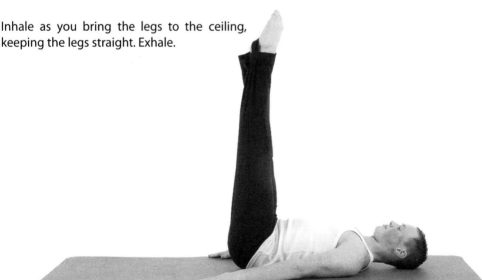

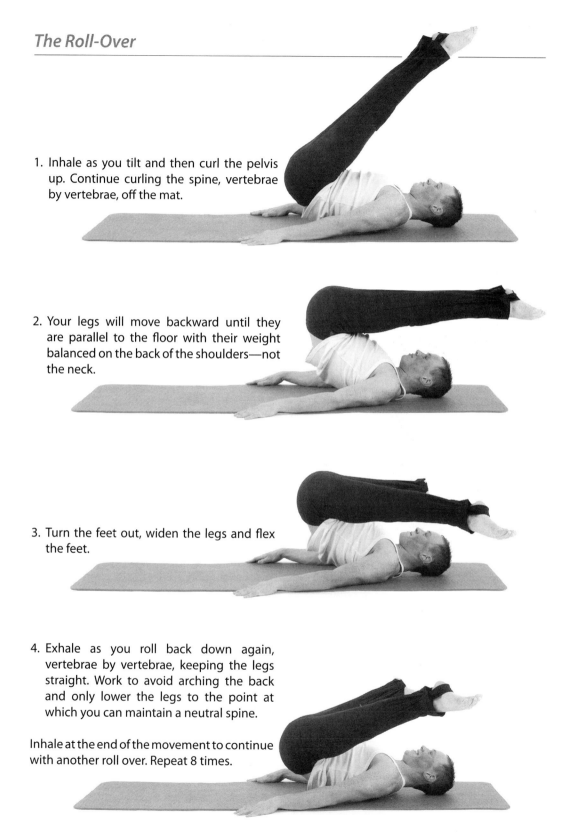

1. Inhale as you tilt and then curl the pelvis up. Continue curling the spine, vertebrae by vertebrae, off the mat.

2. Your legs will move backward until they are parallel to the floor with their weight balanced on the back of the shoulders—not the neck.

3. Turn the feet out, widen the legs and flex the feet.

4. Exhale as you roll back down again, vertebrae by vertebrae, keeping the legs straight. Work to avoid arching the back and only lower the legs to the point at which you can maintain a neutral spine.

Inhale at the end of the movement to continue with another roll over. Repeat 8 times.

Teaser

Teaser is a strength building exercise that requires balance and control as well as the ability to move vertebrae in the spine in a progression. It is a very challenging exercise for the core.

Teaching Points

The teaser requires you to have good length of the hamstrings to achieve full height of the legs during the movement.

Always keep your arms parallel with your legs throughout the movement.

Before you try the teaser be sure that you can control the rocker prep. Next, try to advance the roll back. First, extend one leg away from the body keeping your arms parallel with this extended leg and then roll back so you only have one leg on the floor. Now try extending both legs. Tight hamstrings may limit you at this level. If you can perform this movement you can move to the full teaser.

To Prepare

Sit with your arms by your side and extend your legs in front of you.

Roll back through the spine and lift your legs as you extend them away from the body, bringing the arms up into the air, parallel with the legs.

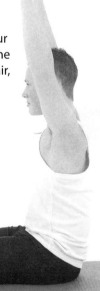

1. Exhale as you roll back up through the spine, keeping the legs extended and the arms parallel to the legs.

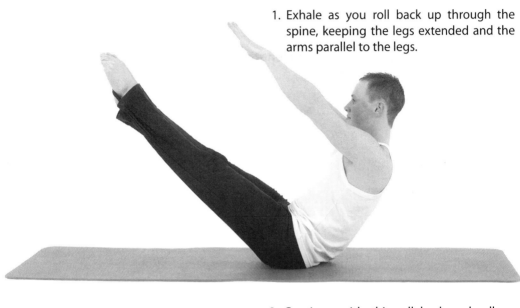

2. Continue with this roll back and roll up action, keeping the legs extended in front of you.

   Repeat 8 times.

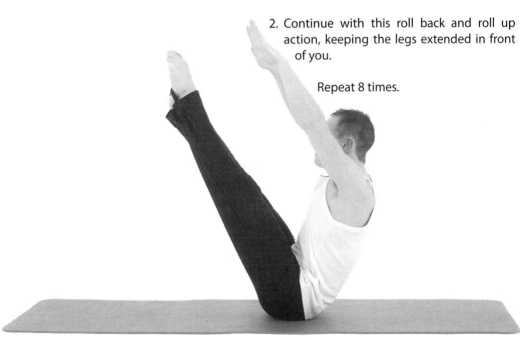

Rolling Back Series

The rolling back exercises will strengthen the deep abdominal muscles—to get the return from the rolling back position. You will also get a massaging effect of the spine; the erector spinae muscles of the back are warmed as they work in a stretched position. This will help ease tension in the back. A final important benefit of this and the other rolling exercises is an improvement in balance.

Teaching Points

The rolling back series, which includes The Seal, Open Leg Rocker and Rolling Like a Ball have been put in the strength section of this book, as they require high levels of abdominal control. From a teaching perspective, however, it is often found that a common fault with this exercise is not being able to initiate the roll back and achieve and hold the "C" curve of the spine. This position requires spine flexibility.

You will need to know that you can achieve the "C" curve position of the spine before you can roll back, or you will throw your head and shoulders back to initiate the movement and will then be unable to return. If your abdominals are not strong enough to bring you back, then you will find yourself flinging your legs to return. First master the rocker prep and the roll back exercise before you try these exercises. It is the tilt of the pelvis that initiates both the roll back and the return. To roll back you must tilt the pelvis backward and to return you must tip the pelvis back to neutral.

The rolling back exercises are often used as a warm down exercise for a matwork program.

Relax the upper body as you perform this movement. If you tense, you will find the rolling movement difficult. Keep the chin tucked into the chest.

Please note that the exercises of the rolling back series are not recommended for anyone with Osteoporosis.

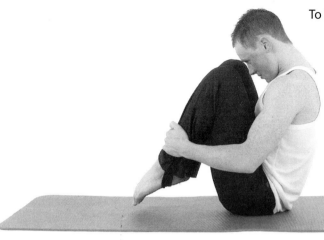

To Prepare

Sit with your knees bent and your heels close to your buttocks. Place your hands on the outside of your ankles and then balance on your sit bones. Bring your feet one inch off of the floor. Your abdominals should be engaged to help with balance. Bring your chin to your chest.

Inhale as you tuck your tailbone under and roll back to your shoulder blades.

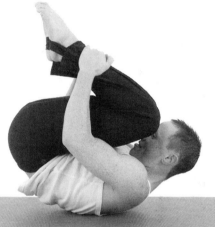

Exhale as you roll back up to the start position.

Repeat up to 8 times.

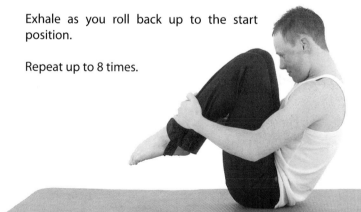

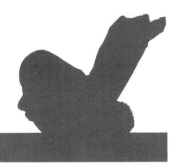

The Seal

To Prepare

Sit tall with your back straight and your knees bent. Your toes should be pointed and touching the floor. Place your hands between your knees and reach around the outside of the ankle with your fingers on the sides of your feet. Push your knees against your arms, just wider than your shoulders and balance with your feet just off the floor. Bring your chin to your chest, look toward your stomach and engage your deep abdominals.

The Seal Movement

1. Inhale as you clap your feet together 3 times, tuck your tailbone under and roll back to your shoulder blades and then repeat the clapping action 3 times.

2. Exhale as you roll back up to the start position and clap 3 times again.

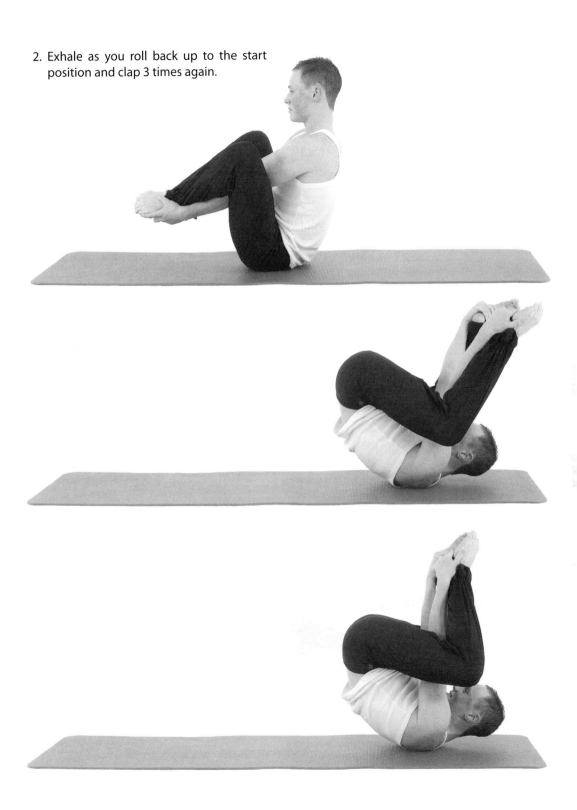

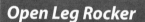

Open Leg Rocker

This is a challenging exercise that requires good flexibility and very supple hamstrings! The abdominals are greatly challenged and the movement requires you to use sequential control between the upper and lower abdominals.

TeachingPoints

Prepare for this exercise with the Open Leg Balance to ensure you have the flexibility and the Rolling Like a Ball to ensure that you understand the rolling back movement. You can then combine the two with the Open Leg Rocker.

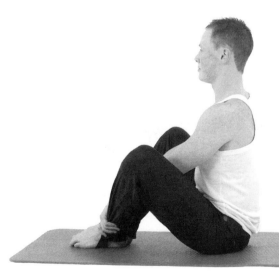

To Prepare

Sit tall with your back straight and your knees bent. Your toes should be pointed and touching the floor. Place your hands between your knees and reach around the outside of the ankles.

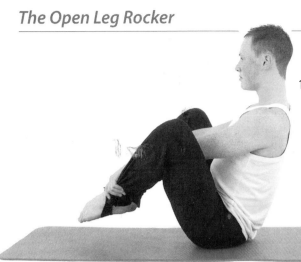

1. Curve your spine into the "C" curve position. Maintaining the height of the back, tighten your abdominals and lift and extend one leg, then the other, so they are shoulder width apart and extended. Balance in this position.

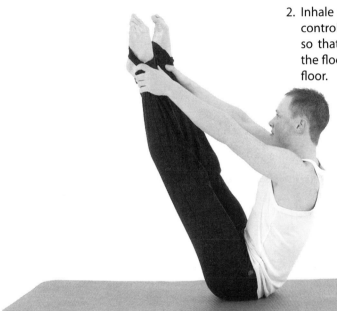

2. Inhale as you initiate the roll back action, controlling with the core muscles. Continue so that the shoulder blades are touching the floor but the head and neck are off the floor.

3. Exhale as you use the abdominals to bring you back to an upright position. Balance here to prepare to repeat the movement.

Repeat up to 4 times.

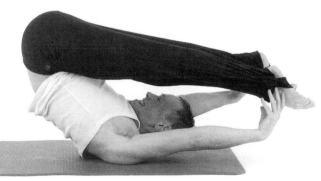

Advanced Pelvic Stability

Shoulder Bridge

This exercise from Joseph Pilates' original Contrology matwork program challenges advanced pelvic stability.

Shoulder bridge works the gluteus maximus muscle, a powerful hip extensor and the hamstring muscles. It also stretches the hip flexor muscles. Taking one leg away challenges the gluteus medius muscle, the main pelvic stabilizer. The core abdominal muscles also work hard to stabilize.

Teaching Points

If you cannot lift the leg without dropping the pelvis on one side, you need to strengthen the gluteus medius muscle with the clam and side kick series. You will then be able to challenge with this advanced level. You must be able to control the bridge with the leg lift exercise before this movement is attempted.

The gluteus maximus muscle is initially targeted with the pelvic tilt and back curl, which is then advanced to the bridge series.

To Prepare

Lie on the floor with your knees bent and your arms by your side. Flatten the small of your back into the floor and lift the tailbone and pelvis so that you have a straight line from your knee to your shoulder.

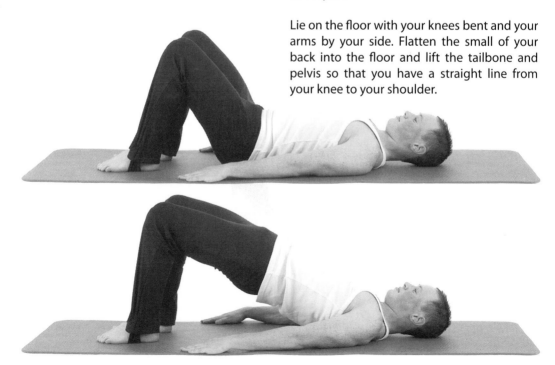

The Full Shoulder Bridge Movement

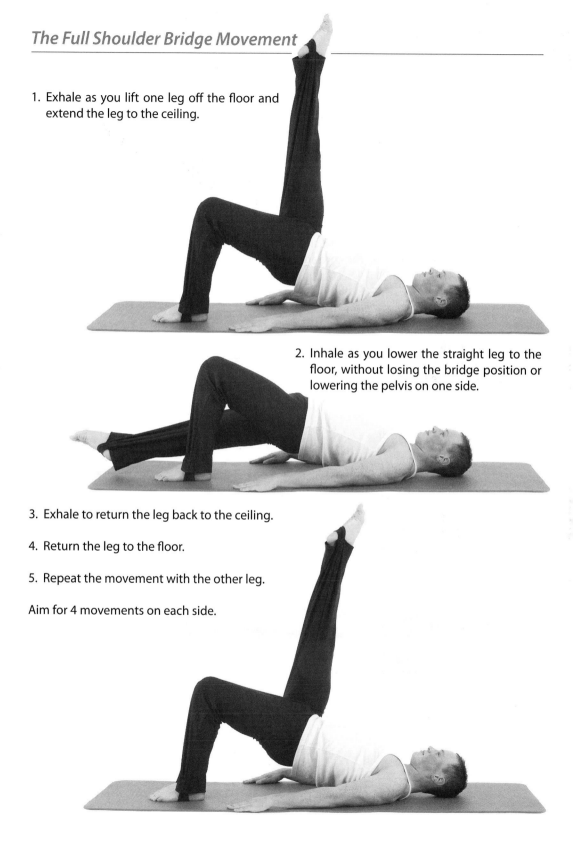

1. Exhale as you lift one leg off the floor and extend the leg to the ceiling.

2. Inhale as you lower the straight leg to the floor, without losing the bridge position or lowering the pelvis on one side.

3. Exhale to return the leg back to the ceiling.

4. Return the leg to the floor.

5. Repeat the movement with the other leg.

Aim for 4 movements on each side.

One Leg Circle

The leg circle exercise focuses on isolating the movers of the hip joint. It is an effective exercise to isolate, strengthen and stabilize the hip joint.

The one leg circle tones and stretches the thigh and improves flexibility of the hip.

Teaching Points

The abdominal muscles work to keep the shoulders and pelvis stable against the movement of the leg. The bigger and faster the leg movements, the harder the abdominals and pelvic stabilizers have to work.

This exercise can be made easier by bending the knee of the moving leg and keeping the circles smaller and slower. You must keep the hips still either side. Bending the supporting knee is a further modification.

Try to keep the shoulders relaxed throughout this movement.

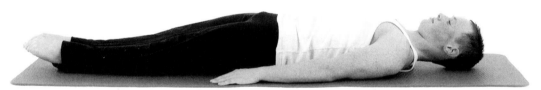

To Prepare

Lie on your back with your hands by your sides and both legs straight. Lift the right leg to the ceiling and point your toe, without arching the lower back and losing neutral spine.

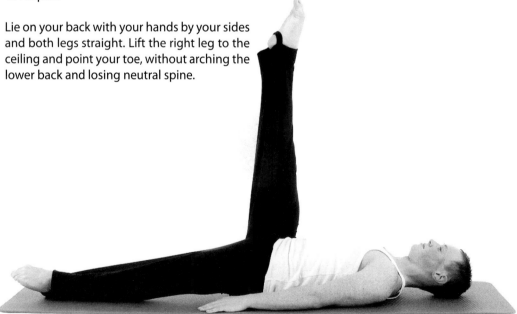

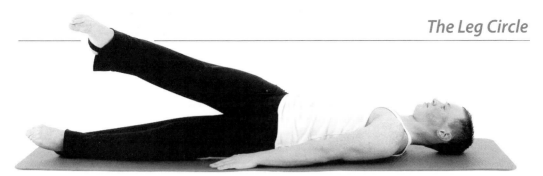

1. Exhale as you lower the leg and bring it over the left thigh. Inhale to bring the leg back up to the ceiling completing a full circle. Continue with this leg for 4 circles. Now change the direction of the circle for 4 further moves.

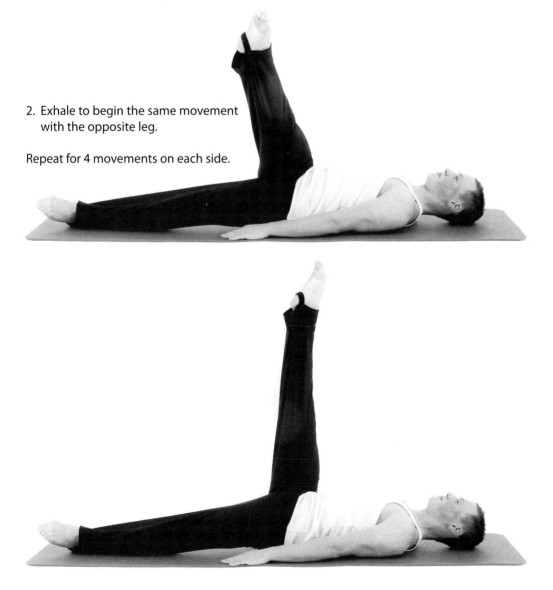

2. Exhale to begin the same movement with the opposite leg.

Repeat for 4 movements on each side.

Side Kick Kneeling

The side kick in kneeling is a pelvic stability exercise that improves balance. Balance requires stability in both the hips and waist and this exercise challenges both.

The oblique muscles work to maintain trunk and pelvic stability throughout this exercise.

Teaching Points

Make sure that you keep your body aligned for this exercise. Don't let the body tip either backward or forward as the leg moves. The movement should be isolated to the hip joint.

Start with small movements and then, as you get stronger, you can increase the swing while still maintaining full control. You will actually feel the gluteus muscles working on both the moving and stabilizing side.

To build the strength required for this exercise, do the side kick series and the clam series to build gluteus medius strength and strengthen the obliques with the criss cross exercise.

To Prepare

Start in an upright kneeling position.

Move to the right side so that your weight is on your right knee only and support your body on your outstretched right arm. Stretch the left leg out to the side in a straight line to the body. Bring your left arm to the side of your head.

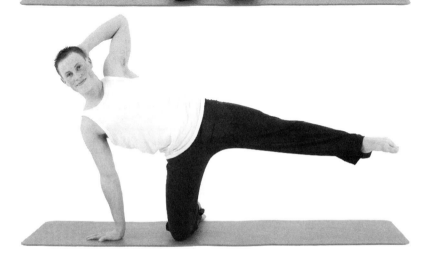

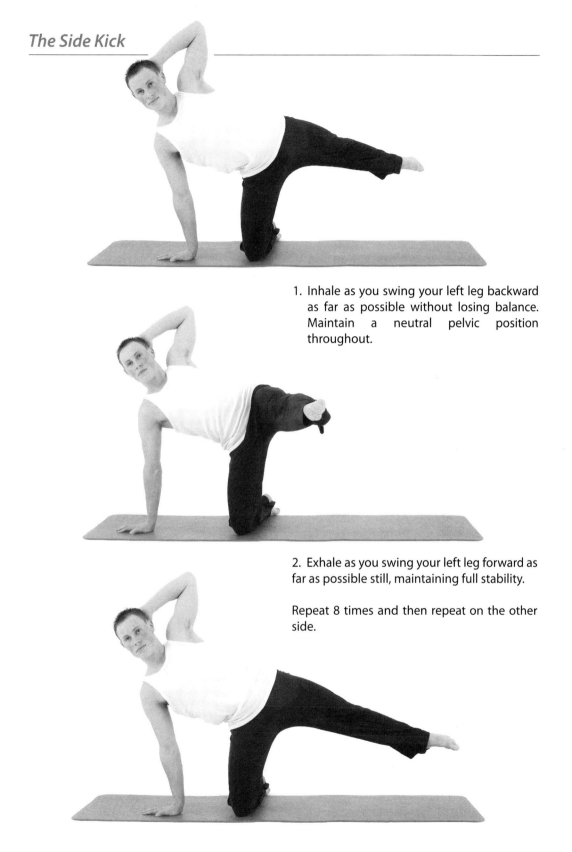

1. Inhale as you swing your left leg backward as far as possible without losing balance. Maintain a neutral pelvic position throughout.

2. Exhale as you swing your left leg forward as far as possible still, maintaining full stability.

Repeat 8 times and then repeat on the other side.

Advanced Scapular Stability

The Push Up

The push up strengthens the rotator cuff muscles of the shoulder. These muscles are important shoulder stabilizers and are often weak in those of us with poor posture.

The push up strengthens the chest, upper arms, shoulders and upper back. It also uses the abdominals to control the movement.

The full press up from standing also stretches the hamstrings, firms the thighs and buttocks and works the back extensor muscles.

Teaching Points

You can make the push up easier by keeping the knees on the floor. Work through the push up prep movements first.

The push up movement should be performed slowly to ensure that you work the right muscles with the correct technique.

Make sure with the movement that you keep your back straight, maintaining neutral spine. You should relax between your shoulder blades and keep your head lengthened and lifted up toward the ceiling.

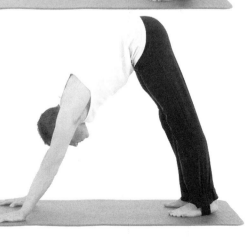

To Prepare

From a standing position, bend forward toward the floor, keeping the lower abdominals in and tightened.

Walk your hands forward so that your legs are extended and your back is straight; your arms will be under your shoulders.

The Push Up

1. Inhale to bend the elbows and lower the body toward the floor. Keep your chin tucked in and your abdominals engaged. Don't tense the upper body and keep your back broad.

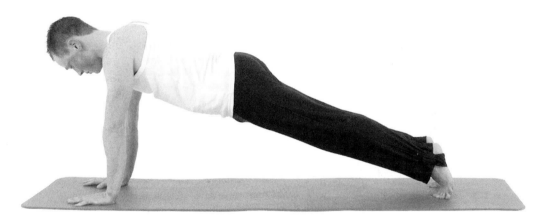

2. Exhale to press back up. Repeat for 8 push ups.

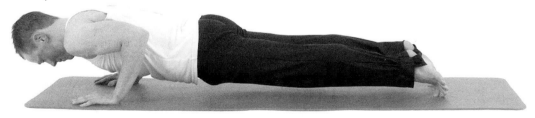

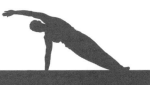

Side Bend

The side bend is an advanced exercise for the oblique muscles. It will lengthen and strengthen the waistline, which is good news for those love handles and spare tires around the mid section!

The side bend also targets the muscles of the arm, shoulder and wrist, building upper body strength.

Teaching Points

Keep the body in alignment for this movement. Do not allow the body to roll either forward or backward.

This movement can be made harder by adding a twist. The twist exercise is in the rehabilitation section for spinal stability.

The sitting or standing side stretch is a much easier version of stretching the same muscles. The obliques can also be targeted by the full criss cross or preparations for the criss cross.

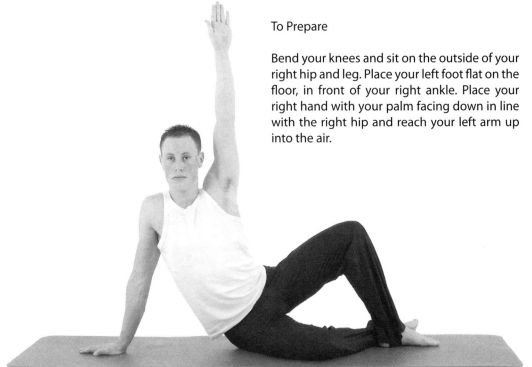

To Prepare

Bend your knees and sit on the outside of your right hip and leg. Place your left foot flat on the floor, in front of your right ankle. Place your right hand with your palm facing down in line with the right hip and reach your left arm up into the air.

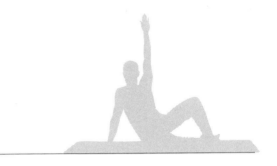

The Side Bend

1. On your next exhalation, engage your core muscles and press down through the right hand to lift your body into a side bend, arching the left arm up over your left ear at the top of the movement. Keep your body in a straight line without dropping in the waist and leaning. Hold this position for between 10 and 30 seconds.

Repeat on the other side.

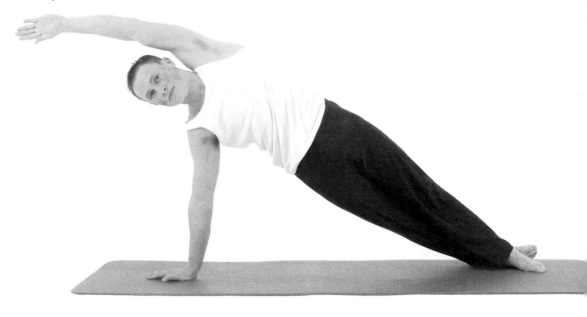

Spine Stretch

The spine stretch is a versatile exercise to increase spinal flexibility. It stretches and eases the strain of tight back muscles, stretches the hamstrings and reinforces good posture.

Teaching Points

If your hamstrings are too tight for you to be able to sit with your legs extended and your back straight, you will need to sit on a foam block or a folded towel. You can perform the movement with bent knees, but you will not get a hamstring stretch.

If you are tight in your hips, you may feel this exercise in the muscle at the front of the top of your thighs. This is especially common if you spend long hours sitting throughout the day. Sitting on a block should help.

To Prepare

Sit with the legs extended straight out in front of you. Keep your back straight and maintain a neutral spine. Point your toes to the ceiling. Put your arms out in front.

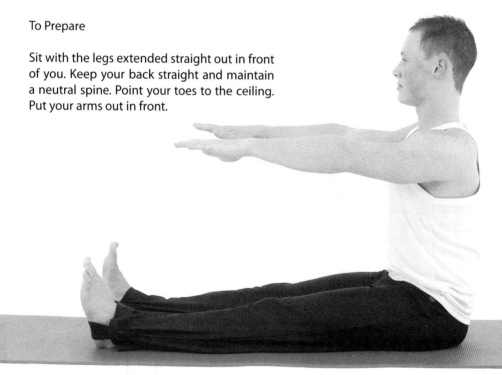

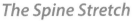

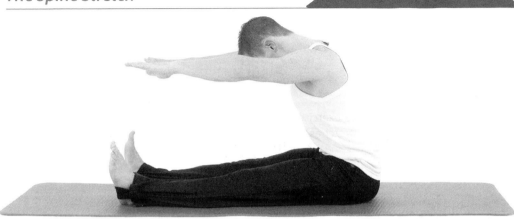

Inhale and round the upper back forward making a deep "C" curve of the spine. Exhale to reach a little further forward. Inhale.

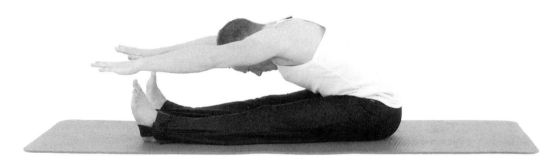

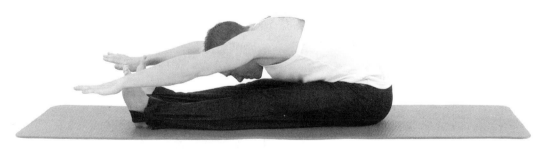

Exhale to return, one vertebrae at a time. Keep your shoulders relaxed throughout.

Repeat 8 times.

The Saw

The saw is a good flexibility exercise that will lengthen the hamstrings, improve spinal rotation and also strengthen the obliques and release tension in the back muscles.

Teaching Points

The emphasis with the saw should be on maintaining a neutral spine and keeping your abdominals engaged throughout. You must not collapse in order to reach toward your toes. It is important to begin with small movements and then increase as your flexibility improves. Remember that quality of movement is of paramount importance with this exercise.

You can sit on a block if necessary to achieve the correct starting position, especially if you have tight hamstrings.

As you reach toward the opposite foot, keep your sitting bone on the floor on the side you are reaching away from.

As you twist, keep your arms stretched to the sides and keep your nose in line with the center of your chest. Only bring one arm forward as you reach for the opposite foot.

The saw movement combines a twist, curve and a reach component. The spine twist will help to improve the rotation of the spine and the spine stretch will help to improve the curve and reach.

To Prepare

Sit tall with your back straight and your legs extended slightly wider than your shoulders. Stretch the arms to the sides. Lift up through the back of the head.

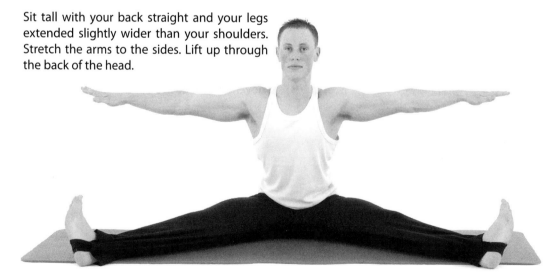

The Saw

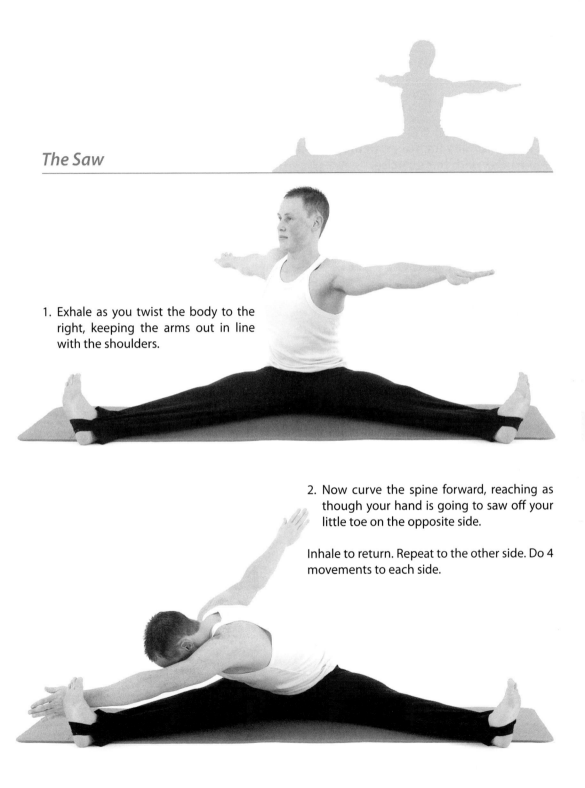

1. Exhale as you twist the body to the right, keeping the arms out in line with the shoulders.

2. Now curve the spine forward, reaching as though your hand is going to saw off your little toe on the opposite side.

Inhale to return. Repeat to the other side. Do 4 movements to each side.

Notes